▲▲▲
Lingam Massage

Lingam Massage

▲▲▲

Awakening Male Sexual Energy

Michaela Riedl and Jürgen Becker

Translated by Nikolas Win Myint

Destiny Books
Rochester, Vermont • Toronto, Canada

Destiny Books
One Park Street
Rochester, Vermont 05767
www.DestinyBooks.com

Destiny Books is a division of Inner Traditions International

Originally published in German under the title *Lingam-Massage: Die Kraft männlicher Sexualität neu erleben* by Hans-Nietsch-Verlag
First U.S. edition published in 2010 by Destiny Books

Library of Congress Cataloging-in-Publication Data
Riedl, Michaela.
  [Lingam Massage. English]
  Lingam massage : awakening male sexual energy / Michaela Riedl and Jürgen Becker ; Translated by Nikolas Win Myint.
     p. cm.
  Includes bibliographical references and index.
  ISBN 978-1-59477-314-3 (pbk.)
  1. Massage. 2. Sexual excitement. 3. Men—Sexual behavior. I. Becker, Jürgen.
II. Myint, Nikolas Win. III. Title.
  RA780.5.R54 2010
  615.8'22081—dc22
                                                                    2009053227

Printed and bound in the United States

10 9 8 7 6 5

Photographs by Bernd Eidenmüller, with assistance from Frank Fleuchaus
Illustrations by Devam Will

Text design and layout by Virginia Scott Bowman
This book was typeset in Garamond Premier Pro and Gill Sans with Torino, Augustea, and Gill Sans as display typefaces

Contents

2 ▲ Energetic and Spiritual Basics 70

4 ▲ The Blessings of Anal and Prostate Massage   158

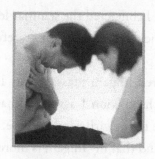

Preface

By Jürgen Becker

It was about one year ago that my partner and I joined a group practicing with Pamela Behnke, a former student of Michaela Riedl and now owner of the "Taste of Touch Center for Sensuality and Joy of Life."* From the first visit, I was struck by the sensitive, loving, and professional way in which Pamela guided us week by week. Contrary to the sexuality that I'd known up to that point, the lingam-yoni massage group was not primarily concerned with erotic stimulation and cosmic orgasms (as pleasant as these might be), but rather with sexual consciousness. In this group I gained not only a completely new relationship to my lingam, but also to my masculinity as a whole.

I sensed then that I was encountering a type of sexuality that was not dependent on hormonal pressure and external stimuli, but one that could nourish and accompany me into my old age. It was this recognition that led me to want to document this wonderful way of sexual self-examination from the male point of view in a book. And it was

*You can learn more about Pamela Behnke from her website: www.taste-of-touch.de

based on this wish that I contacted the seminar leader and author of the book *Yoni Massage*, Michaela Riedl. I am grateful to have knocked on an open door with my proposal.

Before I encountered lingam massage, my lingam was something that had to work. With oblivion I assumed that it was the job of my lingam to give pleasure to my girlfriend and me. Through lingam massage I grew to understand that my lingam is more than just a part of my body: it is a reflection of my relationship to myself and my life force. It is about honoring the man in me. By entering and fostering a loving and conscious relationship with our lingams and our desire, we men are also discovering new ways of dealing with our relationships.

I had never understood why the lingam was revered in Far Eastern traditions; I'd assumed this reverence was due to superstition and tradition. Today I understand that the lingam represents more than just superstition. It is the honoring of male reproductive and creative energy, and also the honoring of masculinity.

This changed relationship to my lingam has also found its expression in my sexuality. It used to be that when I caressed my lingam, I was doing it to satisfy a desire, not to "honor" anything. It was the same when I caressed a yoni; intercourse or the orgasm of my partner were my goals. I have now stopped working toward these goals, and instead touch my lingam or a yoni to honor what it means to be a man or a woman. I remain in the here and now in my touch, and with my hands feel what the lingam and yoni are trying to tell me. I allow them to invite me on a journey in which thoughts, touch, and sensation melt into one.

I now experience an increased awareness of my lingam in everyday life as well, sensing it as a calm strength that was not previously present. Every once in a while I breathe into my lingam and feel its warmth like an oven that comforts me. My lingam, which used to go out into the world, has more and more returned to its home within me. I myself have become the source of my sexual experiences.

For many years I have been moved by the quote of spiritual teacher Barry Long, who said that "there are two ways for the penis to be aroused—through emotion or through love." Only today do I fully understand the meaning of his message in my own body. It is a wonderful feeling for me to be aroused through love and to enjoy it. I share this positive approach to a fulfilled sexuality with other men, women, and couples in my counseling practice, both alone and with my partner.

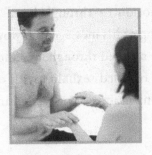

Preface

By Michaela Riedl

When I was about to give my first lingam massage in 1995 I was incredibly excited and surprised by the many ways a lingam can be touched and honored. Up to that point I had not had much experience with male sexuality, and my relationship with the lingam was correspondingly limited.

In the context of my tantric training, I followed the demonstration of lingam massage closely, equipped with notepad and pencil, since as a diligent student I did not want to miss a thing. My thoughts were racing, my pulse quickened, and I became dizzy when faced with the many different massage techniques, since it seemed impossible to remember everything.

When it was my turn, I was comforted by the thought that I would give my best, even if it wasn't perfect. I opened myself to my Shiva and began contact. I looked long and deeply into my partner's eyes and suddenly felt very clearly that I was faced with someone who was not expecting a perfect massage, but a man who simply wanted to be touched, honored, and loved.

The massage began. I gave my best, but my Shiva did not become erect during the entire massage. My thoughts raced: "What am I doing wrong?" "Is he not enjoying my touch?" "What I'm doing must feel terrible—I hope nobody notices how bad I am at this!"

Afterward, we held each other and talked. He assured me that my touch had felt good, but that he had been too excited to get an erection. For me as a woman it was completely new that a man could enjoy having his lingam touched without getting an erection. It was good to speak with him, and to let go of my fixed ideas of what and how sex had to be.

Since then I have asked men many questions and know now that many of my assumptions about male sexuality and masculinity were never correct. However, it's not an easy thing to change them, and I have found that old prejudices and views are powerful, anchored deep within us and rising to the surface as soon as we feel insecure. It is a love of humanity that invites us again and again to let go of old prejudices and misconceptions, and allows us to be open to the unknown and to the present. Nourishing sexuality requires safety, acceptance, understanding, and love. This is as true for men as it is for women.

Just like women, men need an encouraging environment to develop their sexuality. This includes not only the external conditions, but also a relaxed and accepting partner—who does not have to be "perfect," but who does have to be loving and empathetic.

In our AnandaWave trainings and seminars about yoni and lingam massage, which I co-lead with Gitta Arntzen, we continue to address the question of how it is possible to teach different qualities of touch without leading to unrealistic expectations or a limiting focus on performance. And again we only have one answer to that question—it is a love of what we do, and who we do it with. It is something that all of us are learning—that we do our best in a massage, even if again and again we encounter things that don't immediately "work." This requires humor, love, and tolerance.

Because our ingrained prejudices do not disappear from one day to the next, understanding sexuality is by necessity a process, not an event. But life is not as hard or as serious as we often think. If we are able to laugh with love when a child learns to walk and falls down clumsily every once in a while, we should be equally able to laugh with love at life and sexuality.

Yoni and lingam massages offer couples a wonderful opportunity to explore themselves and each other with humor, in a clearly defined framework, without prejudice or expectations. The experiences and knowledge gained in this way can then be playfully applied during lovemaking. In this way, couples learn a great deal about themselves, since they have the opportunity to experience themselves in a new way, independent of the needs and expectations of their partners. We can only be good lovers when we know ourselves and our own needs.

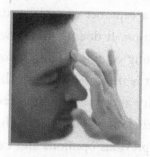

Introduction

The English language does not have a reverent word for the lingam: unfortunately, neither *penis,* nor *cock,* nor *dick* even begins to reflect the significance that the lingam can have for a man. Instead, these words demonstrate that we do not have a conscious, loving relationship with this part of our bodies.

Although all of these words may refer to the same body part, a lingam is different than a cock. Our words evoke a certain spirit, and when we ask if our loved one wants us to revere his lingam, this imparts a different meaning than when we ask if we should rub his cock. Thus, the choice of the word *lingam* is a conscious one, because historically it has conveyed reverence, respect, attention, and loving touch. By referring to other states of energy and consciousness, the word thus makes it easier for us to describe lingam massage.

As we will see, lingam massage is a holy and healing act, even while it involves sexuality. It expresses a loving and selfless attention to the lingam that may at first seem foreign or unusual. The lingam is honored and caressed with differentiated movements that are filled with tenderness and acceptance. This combination can allow a man to strengthen his sense of masculinity, or even to "surf" on an ocean of heightened sensations.

The discovery and acceptance of male sexual strength is independent of potency or erection. It doesn't matter whether the recipient of a lingam massage is young or old, potent or not, sexually experienced or inexperienced. What is important is his willingness to explore this new part of his sexuality and to consciously feel it. Sexual consciousness begins with accepting oneself as one is. This requires a journey of discovery in which all previous opinions and experiences are set aside, allowing us to experience ourselves in a new way.

What we can discover on this journey is a new way of life. We discover our masculinity, freedom, independence from external stimuli, and ability to love. A man who knows himself and his lingam has a deeper relationship with himself, and knows what is true for him and what is not. The conscious contact with one's masculinity—the goal of lingam massage—allows men to build a bridge to the feminine without resorting to crybaby or macho posturing. Men no longer need to protect themselves against female emotions or seduction, but are instead able to be in loving and lustful contact with the feminine.

At the same time, lingam massage remains a mystery. The Zen concept of "beginner's mind" conveys the ability to experience something without prejudice, as if we were encountering it for the first time, like a child marveling at a flower. If we can approach lingam massage with the same openness, despite all our knowledge, then every individual massage will bring new wonders. Free of judgment and comparison, we will experience the unique miracle of recognizing every moment as a new expression of creation itself.

We are feeling beings. We all seek to be happy and search for the source of happiness. This is what makes us human and what connects all of us. Lingam massage is a step in this direction.

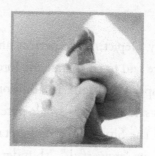

1
Male Sexuality

In the lingam, see the beauty of solidified gold,
the steadiness of the Himalayas,
the tenderness of a growing leaf,
the life-giving strength of the sun,
and the stimulation of its sparkling jewels!

LINGA PURANA

THE LINGAM AS SYMBOL

The word *lingam* refers to the innermost core of masculinity. It comes from Sanskrit, the holy language of India, and means "pillar of light," "wall of light," "stick of jade," and "lotus sword." In India, the lingam is revered as an expression of Shiva's clarity, able to penetrate the fog of illusion—false ideas and beliefs. The lingam symbolizes the fine sword that differentiates between the true and the false and between our own creative energy and the energy of creation.

Two-colored stones found in central western India's Narmada River are taken as representatives of the lingam in India. They are seen as holy and are shaped by hand into a typical oval form and polished. The shape of the stone symbolizes male energy, while the reddish brown segments symbolize female energy. Depicting the perfect union of heart-connected life energy, the stones are said to regenerate life force and to have a harmonizing effect on body, spirit, and soul. In addition, wearing such a stone or meditating on one is said to increase male potency and stamina.

What Indians call the Shiva lingam, Tibetans refer to as *vajra* or *dorje,* meaning "hard" or "powerful," "thunder stroke" or "scepter of diamonds." The vajra is associated with terms like *unbreakable, indestructible,* and *insurmountable.* It is seen as the symbol of the highest spiritual power, against which nothing is immune. The vajra spirit is seen as a state of enlightenment: pure and hard as a diamond, able to cut through all material things without suffering damage to itself. In this way, the vajra is the visible symbol of those who have within themselves the highest spiritual powers, including stamina, goal-orientation, creative energy, the ability to create structure, and the willingness to sacrifice in the pursuit of larger goals.

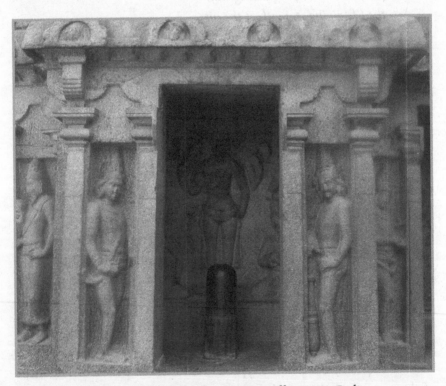

Fig. 1.1. A Shiva lingam in Mamallapuram, India

Ancient tribes used to see magic in the lingam's ability to become hard. Today, we no longer have the same appreciation for nature's miracles. But is it not a wonderful spectacle when the lingam rises? And doesn't an erect lingam recall the scepter of a king or the wand of a magician?

Maori magicians place a hand on the lingam when casting a spell to draw on its supernatural power. Ancient books describe the practice of placing a hand on the lingam or testicles when making an oath, to express sincerity. In some parts of Morocco this practice continues into the present.

Many traditions see the male aspect of god as conveying steadiness and eternity, while the female aspect of god is its transformative power. In this way, honoring the lingam creates a connection between us and eternity.

Chinese Taoist teachings refer to the lingam as the "jade stick" or "carnelian bird." Since ancient times, the Chinese have viewed the lingam and yoni as important parts of the body that required as much touch, care, and love as all the other parts. Lingam massage is inspired by old Taoist teachings. It is one of the deepest internal experiences a man can have, simultaneously healing and energizing.

The lingam is every man's "magic wand." But, like a plant or a pet, it requires loving care to maintain its powers. If we give it respect, love, and touch, the lingam will teach us a new form of love and creative energy. In our culture, however, the lingam is often "used" as a penetrating or satisfying organ, rather than deeply loved.

During hundreds of years of influence from the church and its dogmas, sexuality was devalued, as were women and their powers of secret knowledge. This made it increasingly difficult for feminine power to honor masculine power and its lingam. Men lost their consciousness of the lingam as an organ of love, and began to use it with a fixation on the personal goal of achieving orgasm. This narrow focus often led women to fear the lingam, and prevented them from recognizing it as an enriching part of their sexual experience. Thus, the lingam has rarely received the love that it deserves.

EXPLORING THE LINGAM

An increasing number of people, women as well as men, now understand that the lingam should be appreciated as an "organ of love." They
stop reducing the penis to an "organ of function" that is expected to
grow erect and produce orgasms, and recognize that our interactions
with the lingam are about more than getting it up, in, and out. Instead,
lingam massage increases our consciousness of our entire being. It is a
new way of loving and of living.

Before we review the different phases of lingam massage, it is important to understand the lingam's varied anatomy. Most of it is visible—
the shaft, glans, foreskin, frenulum, urethra opening, scrotum, and
perineum—while other parts such as the prostate, testicles, and rectum
can be felt but not seen.

If you choose, you can now take some time to explore your lingam.
Create a pleasant, warm room and make sure that you won't be disturbed
for the next two hours. You will need a mirror and some lubricant.

Alternatively, you can explore your lingam along with your partner; this will allow you to share your feelings, sensations, and thoughts,
while allowing your partner to be in contact with your lingam without
a specific goal in mind. If you do this, avoid evaluating, commenting, or
discussing anything, and make sure there is enough trust between the
two of you to avoid any feelings of shame.

Whether alone or with a partner, begin the exploration of your
lingam with love and joyful, sensual expectations. If you are standing
in front of a large mirror and looking at the front of your body, you can
see your hairy pubic hill, which this book will refer to as the lingam
hill. If you are exploring your partner's lingam, ask him to allow you to
look at and touch his lingam.

The Lingam

The shaft of the penis begins below the lingam hill. It ends in the protruding "head" or glans (*glans penis*) that sits on the shaft like a round

cap. The skin around the shaft feels soft and movable; the skin of the glans is usually significantly redder than that of the shaft. If the man is uncircumcised, the glans is covered by the foreskin. Carefully pulling back the foreskin, you will see and feel that the skin between shaft and glans is thinner and more sensitive than it is elsewhere. At the front of the glans, the frenulum connects it to the underside of the penis.

When the penis is not erect, the glans is very sensitive, especially to the touch. When the penis is erect, the sensitivity of the glans decreases. The nerve endings of the frenulum are also very sensitive, which makes careful touching of this spot, especially when erect, very pleasurable for men.

To the left and right sides of the frenulum, as well as immediately below the edge of the glans, is the so-called "male clitoris"—an area that roughly corresponds to the female clitoris. This delicate area is often not explored among men, since ejaculation and orgasm are usually initiated primarily by rubbing the foreskin across the glans. While the male clitoris corresponds to the female clitoris in many ways, its orgasmic signals are more subtle in men than in women. If this area is massaged and caressed well, it can become a source of great sexual pleasure for men.

At the tip of the glans is the opening of the urethra, which has an impressive dual function: both semen—a mix of secretions from the testicles, seminal vesicles, prostate, and Cowper's glands—and urine from the bladder are excreted here, though never at the same time.

The Testicles

Below the lingam and connected to the lower part of the body is the scrotum, which in its left and right sides contains the two egg-shaped testicles. In an evolutionary sense, the scrotum corresponds to the female outer labia, while the testicles correspond to the female ovaries. The testicles, especially in a non-aroused state, are very sensitive to pain through pressure or squeezing. But when held gently or lightly caressed, they can be a source of great pleasure, especially if the lingam is caressed at the same time.

A good way of touching the testicles is to make a ring with thumb and index finger around the scrotum above the testicles—taking care not to squeeze them. Many men find this "testicle ring" very stimulating, and it often increases an erection. When releasing the testicle ring, take a moment to feel the spermatic cords between your fingers. You can also gently unfold the skin of the scrotum and give it a light massage. The gentle touching, rubbing, and pulling of the testicles stimulates testosterone production and increases sperm count.

While some men find testicle massage very pleasurable, others do not enjoy it. It takes some sensitivity to understand what touch is pleasurable to your partner and what is not. If you are massaging your partner's testicles, pay attention to his signals—moaning and "yes" sounds tell you to continue, silence shows that it is not arousing, while small, non-pleasure noises, headshaking, or gestures indicate that it is unpleasant.

Perineum, Prostate, and the "Point of a Million Pieces of Gold"

The following exploration requires a small, handheld mirror. Even better, crouch above a slightly larger mirror, which will allow you to use both hands to explore the area below your testicles.

Between the anus and scrotum is the perineum, which is extremely important for lovemaking and male desire. Using a finger to explore the perineum, begin by feeling the bump that forms the root of the lingam, located immediately behind the testicles. A little further toward the anus is the "point of a million pieces of gold," a soft area into which you can press your finger. Behind this, on the inside of the body, is the prostate, and this is the spot from which it can be felt externally and massaged. Most men and women are surprised when they discover how receptive the prostate is to sexual stimulation.

The prostate is a gland about the size of a chestnut. It is located immediately above the perineum in the center of the pelvis, directly behind the pubic bone. Much like the female G-spot, stimulation of the prostate can cause deep and sustained emotions during male orgasm.

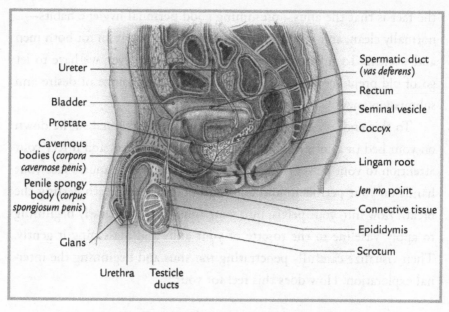

Ureter

Bladder

Prostate

Cavernous
bodies (*corpora
cavernose penis*)

Penile spongy
body (*corpus
spongiosum penis*)

Glans

Urethra Testicle
ducts

Spermatic duct
(*vas deferens*)

Rectum

Seminal vesicle

Coccyx

Lingam root

Jen mo point

Connective tissue

Epididymis

Scrotum

Fig. 1.2. The anatomy of the lingam

Prostate orgasms connect men with their receptive sides, while lingam orgasms tend to connect men more with their dynamic strength.

The Anus

After we have explored the penis and all visible areas of the male genitals, let us explore a less visible and more "forbidden" part of the body, the anus.

Because of its proximity to the prostate and the multitude of sensitive nerve endings there, the anus is a highly erogenous zone for men. However, many men have very little experience, if any, with touch and stimulation of it, in large part because this area continues to be the subject of many taboos, and is often considered dirty and smelly. Among some men, this is mixed with a fear of homosexuality. They do not want to become the penetrated "female."

Of course, it is important to keep the anus clean to avoid the transmission of bacteria. But if it was meant simply for excretion, why would the anus be so sensitive and sexually receptive? Although it is a common misconception that it is perverse or dirty to pay attention to the anus, the fact is that the anus—presuming good personal hygiene habits—is normally clean, and it is an important area of exploration for both men and women. To fully experience its pleasures, however, we have to let go of old prejudice and shame and approach this source of desire and submission anew.

To this end, try the following exercise: preferably naked, lie down on your bed in a comfortable position. Close your eyes and direct your attention to your pelvic floor, and particularly to your anus. Place your hands on your perineum and anus and take a deep breath, letting the breath flow into your pelvis, into your anus. Visualize slowly beginning to apply Vaseline to the rosette of your anus and massaging it gently. Then visualize carefully penetrating the anus and beginning the internal exploration. How does this feel for you?

THE ANATOMY OF
MALE SEXUAL ORGANS

When men think of their masculinity, their thoughts often go straight to that wonderful, energetic, and powerful organ—the penis. This is not surprising, since it is the most noticeable manifestation of masculinity.

As the sociologist Dieter Duhm wrote: "With nothing are men as closely identified than with their penis and its behavior. It is man's pride or downfall, his belonging or non-belonging in the group of men, his connection to the world of women, his passport and measuring stick."

For many of us, male sexuality is still a map with many blank spots that remain undiscovered. For the benefit of men and women alike, the adventure of discovering masculinity can begin.

About the Size of the Lingam

Every lingam is wonderfully unique and different from others in its size and appearance. The length of the penis varies depending on the situation: when a man is afraid or has just been in cold water, his penis can shrink to become almost invisible. When he is aroused, it can grow to its full size.

The size of a non-erect penis gives little indication of its maximum size. There are lingams that are large when at rest, but barely grow when erect (this is called a low "swell factor"), while there are other penises that double in size during erection.

In this context, it is important to note that there are also very different yonis. It can happen that a large lingam may hit a woman's cervix and cause pain, while a small lingam may not fully fill a woman's vagina. But any lingam is large enough to be sexually stimulating, especially for G-spot orgasms, since the G-spot is only 2.5 to 7.5 centimeters inside the yoni. Moreover, there are positions in which the man enters the yoni especially deeply or less so, which allows couples to balance their physical features. We also know that the inside of the yoni swells up when aroused, surrounding the penis tightly, meaning that there is sufficient friction even with a small lingam. Finally, lingam and yoni adjust to each other in shape and size through repeated contact.

Many men falsely think their penises are too small. Older men may complain that their penis has shrunk in recent years, while men who have gained weight complain about fat that covers part of the penis and makes it appear smaller. But these complaints distract from the important facts: more important than size is that lingam and yoni are in loving contact and together carry out the dance of lovers. The size of the penis has nothing to do with a man's strength, and shouldn't be a matter of concern. For most women, the erotic tension between lovers is much more important than the size of the lingam.

Erectile Tissue

The penis is made up primarily of different kinds of erectile tissue—specifically, two parallel columns called the *corpora cavernose penis,* or "cavernous bodies," and the single penile spongy body—the *corpus spongiosum penis*—which contains the urethra. Both of these erectile tissues are composed of many pool-shaped blood vessels within a sponge-like

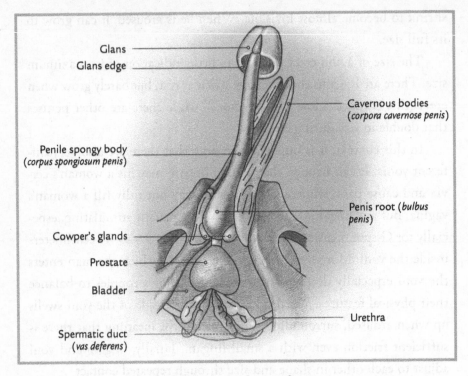

Glans
Glans edge
Cavernous bodies
(*corpora cavernose penis*)
Penile spongy body
(*corpus spongiosum penis*)
Penis root (*bulbus penis*)
Cowper's glands
Prostate
Bladder
Urethra
Spermatic duct
(*vas deferens*)

Fig. 1.3. The male erectile tissue

base that can take in blood and swell, thus causing an erection. When erect, erectile tissues contain about eight to ten times (!) as much blood as they do when not erect.

Although there are no muscles in the penis that are directly visible, individual blood vessels in the erectile tissue are enveloped in muscle cells and connective tissue. The individual vessels look like small corkscrews; they stretch during erection, making the penis grow. The erectile tissue contains the penis arteries and also nerves, which transmit information through electric impulses to the surrounding tissue. The penis itself is linked to the abdominal wall and the pubic bone by two muscles, *m. ischiocavernosi* and *m. bulbosspongioses*.

The spongy body of the penis (the *corpus spongiosum penis* mentioned above) surrounds the urethra and at one end becomes the head, or glans penis. The far end of this tissue grows like an onion bulb and forms the root of the lingam. The spongy body consists mainly of expand-able hollow areas that fill with blood when the lingam becomes erect, but which remain soft and flexible. When the penis is erect, this tissue contains about 10 percent of its total blood volume. The corresponding female tissue is not only the clitoris, as is often assumed because of the visible similarities, but the entire area around the female urethra—the *glans vulvae,* which extends into the vagina entrance immediately below the opening of the urethra.[1]

The erectile tissues of the penis shaft, the *corpora cavernose penis,* are primarily responsible for making the penis stiff during erection. A thin elastic wall partially separates the two columns, which run along parallel tracks from the pelvic floor (the penis root) to the glans. During erection, these columns contain 90 percent of the total blood volume of the penis. In contrast to the spongy body tissue, the cavernous bodies are also enveloped by a dense tissue layer, called the *tunica albuginea.* When the spaces fill with blood during erection, this dense layer tenses and the erectile tissue become hard, making the lingam stiff.

Thank you, *corpora cavernose.*

The cavernous bodies receive the blood supply that hardens the lingam through two pairs of arteries. These arteries run along the inside of the tissue in a snakelike formation, which has many small, tightly branched arteries originating from it. When these small arteries close off their empty spaces, blood flow in the tissue is reduced; blood flows back through the veins, and the lingam loses its erection. The erection is thus caused by the opening of the small arteries (which I will call "inflow" arteries for simplicity's sake), and a corresponding closing of the veins, which reduces the outward flow of blood.

Usually, the inflow arteries are tight and the muscles tense, which prevents blood from filling the cavernous bodies. However, when sex-ual stimuli of any kind reach a man's brain while he is relaxed, they will stimulate nerve impulses that travel from the brain to the penis nerves via the spinal cord. At the nerve endings, various neurotrans-mitter enzymes are released in increasing quantities as the perceived stimuli continue. This leads to an expansion of the blood vessels and a relaxation of the muscles in the erectile tissues. The inflow arteries of the lingam are allowed to open and blood enters the erectile tissue. The speed of blood flow doubles and the tissues swell with blood.

The removal of blood is regulated by the veins of the penis. When the penis is flaccid, the vein tissue is open, allowing an easy return of blood from the penis to the heart. As a man becomes aroused, the vein tissue tightens, reducing the return of blood to a trickle, and increasing the volume of the erectile tissue by a factor of three or four. The lingam grows erect.

When the inflow arteries close off their empty spaces, the flow of blood to the erectile tissue is reduced, the blood returns directly into the veins, and the lingam goes flaccid. The formula is thus very simple: erection means a large blood inflow, and little outflow. Flaccidity means a large blood outflow, with little inflow.

This is very important information for sexual awareness, since it makes clear that the blood that is critical for an erection comes not from muscle strength in the penis, but from a relaxation of the inflow

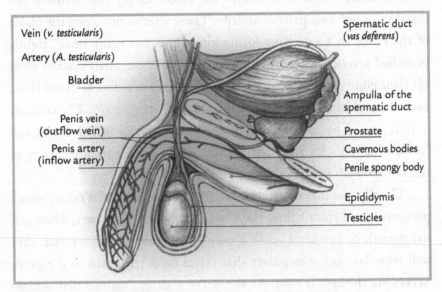

Fig. 1.4. The blood supply of the lingam

arteries. That is why relaxation is an important factor in achieving strong and lasting erections!

The Urethra

The penile spongy body surrounds the urethra, which is responsible for the transport of urine and, during ejaculation, of semen. The urethra begins at the lower end of the bladder, runs across the prostate, the pelvic floor, and the spongy body, before ending in the opening of the glans. Urine can only exit through the small opening at the tip of the penis when the penis is not erect, which is why urine and semen do not flow out simultaneously.

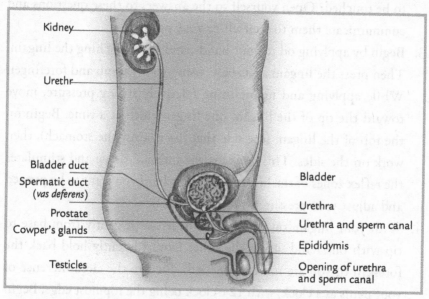

Kidney

Urethr

Bladder duct

Spermatic duct
(*vas deferens*)

Prostate

Cowper's glands

Testicles

Bladder

Urethra

Urethra and sperm canal

Epididymis

Opening of urethra
and sperm canal

Fig. 1.5. The urethra and sperm canal

▲ Massaging the Lingam Shaft

This massage can easily be done alone, and the instructions that follow are directed to the solo practitioner. However, they can also be adapted for a partner. Whether you are by yourself or working with a partner, the first step is to find a comfortable room that is warm and protected against intrusions and surprises.

1. Before beginning a massage of the lingam, make sure that your whole body receives loving touch. Even if you are alone, begin by touching and caressing your whole body. If you are working with a partner, your partner can carry out a full-body massage (see page 127) as an introduction.

2. Undress completely and lie down on your back. Rub your hands against each other until they are warm, then place your left hand on your heart (or on the heart of the man you are massaging) and your right hand on your lingam (or on the lingam of your partner). Listen closely to your heart and lingam and establish contact. What are you feeling? How is your lingam? How do you want your lingam to be touched? Open yourself to the answers to these questions and communicate them to yourself or your partner.

3. Begin by applying oil to your hands, and then touching the lingam. Then press the lingam at its base, using your thumb and forefinger. While applying and maintaining relatively strong pressure, move toward the tip of the lingam one finger-width at a time. Begin on the top of the lingam (the side that lies against the stomach), then work on the sides. This awakens the internal tissue and stimulates the reflex zones of the lingam. Feel how hard you want to be pressed and adjust your pressure or tell your partner.

4. With your lingam on your stomach, stroke it gently from base to tip with one hand, using the other hand to gently hold back the foreskin (if you are not circumcised). Picture the circumference of your penis as a clock, with 12 o'clock being the topmost edge. Begin by stroking at 12 o'clock from base to tip, then at 1 o'clock from base to tip, and so on, continuing until you have returned to the 12 o'clock position. At the 5, 6, and 7 o'clock positions, your hand will be wrapped all the way around your lingam. Does the touch feel different depending on the position of your hand? Try to feel the difference, remain mentally present, and make a conscious effort to enjoy each touch. It is not important whether the lingam is erect or not at this point. If you are erect, pay attention to the course of your

erection and slow down or stop touching yourself if you feel you are getting close to an orgasm. If you are doing this exercise with a partner, communicate with him or her about your preferences and your state of arousal. You will be able to enjoy the massage more fully if you do not ejaculate at this point.

5. Now stroke your hand across your lingam in the other direction; move down from the glans to the testicles and perineum, using your other hand to spread energy throughout your body—for example stroking from one knee across the perineum and back to the other knee, or giving your stomach a little massage. Allow the sexual energy to flow from your hips to every part of your being. Feel every stroke. Breathe, and give in to spontaneous movements of your body. If you are giving a massage to a partner, sit on his right side during this exercise, with your face toward his feet. Distribute the erotic energy throughout his body.

6. Next take your lingam between the flat palms of your hands. (If you are giving a lingam massage to someone else, do this while sitting at your partner's right side. When you take his lingam between your palms, your fingers will be pointing toward his feet.) Slide your hands up and down the lingam, varying your speed and strength. Ask your partner how he likes to be touched. This is usually a very intense and arousing exercise. If you like, massage yourself (or your partner) until just before the point of no return. As the receiving partner, feel your arousal and use your breathing to distribute the erotic energy throughout your body. Give clear signals so your partner can stop before you orgasm.

7. If the lingam is standing upright, you can roll it back and forth between your hands, as if you were rubbing a piece of wood to make fire. This creates strong friction, so use plenty of oil. Keep changing between this stroke and the previous one. This can create a surprising fire that can build vitality and excitement.

8. Massage down to the base and up again to the tip. Use your whole hand to envelop the lingam and stroke it from the base all the way

to the tip, pushing the foreskin over the head. Repeat this stroke, starting again from the base and massaging all the way upward, allowing the phallic energy to rise to the sky. After a few upward strokes, continue the massage in the opposite direction, with both hands enveloping the lingam and alternating as they glide from top to bottom along the shaft. In this way, return the phallic energy to the root. Continue this for as long as it feels good. If you are receiving this massage, try to feel each movement. What stage are you at in your arousal? Be present and continue taking deep breaths.

9. Next hold your hands around the lingam as if in prayer, and glide them up and down. (If you are massaging a partner, sit opposite him.) You can also do this using only one hand, and use the other hand to distribute energy across the body. Whether you're massaging yourself or a partner, allow sufficient time after each phase of the massage for relaxation.

The Glans

After you have thoroughly explored the lingam shaft, it is now time to continue with the glans, the foreskin, the edge of the glans, and the frenulum. These parts of the penis are among the strongest erogenous zones for men. But as noted before, they appreciate only mild to medium stimulation on a non-erect lingam.

The glans is in many ways the crown of the lingam. It is a very sensitive part that is home to many nerve endings, including a main nerve—*nervus dorsalis penis*—that runs across the top of the spongy body. These nerves are connected directly with the brain and transmit information about the state of arousal, erection, and when the time comes, ejaculation.

The glans consists of the glans edge (*corona glandis*) and the glans neck (*collum glandis*), which connect the glans with the lingam shaft. The topmost layer of skin on the glans is very thin—especially among men who are not circumcised—and home to a number of free nerve endings that can register even the smallest stimuli. Some men have many small protruding spots around the edge of the glans, called *hirsuties papillaris*. These are completely normal—not a sign of any illness or a lack of personal hygiene.

While the shaft of the penis can be freely touched, the glans requires great care. Whether a touch is perceived as pleasant or unpleasant is largely related to how it is done, and how relaxed the giving and receiving partners are.

The Foreskin

The whole penis is covered by skin that is made up of fat-free, very loose connective tissue, which is highly flexible and expandable. This allows the skin to adjust to the different sizes of the lingam during erection, and also allows us to stimulate the lingam by moving this skin up and down. The skin that covers the glans is called the foreskin (or prepuce). It is connected to the penis directly underneath the glans, supported by a strip of foreskin called the frenulum, which prevents the foreskin from slipping back all the way.

The area to the left and right of the frenulum, below the glans on the bottom of the lingam (the side that faces the testicles in a non-erect state) is called the foreskin sheet. There are a number of glands in this area that secrete fluids, and it is important for men to regularly wash the area around the frenulum, otherwise white, smelly protein deposits can form here.

The foreskin sheet and the edge of the glans are part of the shaft's erectile tissue, and correspond to the female clitoris. A good massage in this area is very pleasurable for men.

The foreskin itself corresponds to the hood of the female clitoris, and serves to protect the sensitive glans against strong friction and injuries. It also keeps the glans tender and moist. The foreskin consists of two layers of skin—the outer and inner foreskin. The outer skin looks just like the rest of the skin around the penis, while the inner foreskin is a mucous membrane, similar to the skin inside the mouth. These two layers are not tightly grown together, but can move against one another. They contain

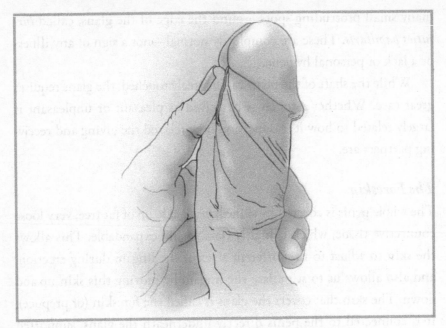

Fig. 1.6. Massaging the "male clitoris"

many nerve endings, which are especially concentrated at the very tip.

Normally, the foreskin can be easily pulled back from the glans, and during erections this happens automatically. While direct stimulation of the glans is often felt as rough or unpleasant, men generally enjoy it when the foreskin rubs across the glans. In fact, this is a popular form of masturbation. Unfortunately, men often restrict themselves to this one masturbation technique, which can increase the incidence of premature ejaculation.[2]

One of the benefits of lingam massage is that it enables men to expand their experience of arousal and sensuality beyond a few "tried and true" techniques. This promotes a more mature relationship between a man and his penis, makes him a better and more enduring lover.

Circumcision

Many men are circumcised; some for religious reasons, and others for cultural or medical reasons. Whether a man is circumcised or not does not make a big difference to his skill as a lover, since both options are equally well suited to satisfying the owner and his partner.

Proponents of circumcision point out that the procedure reduces the risk of penis cancer, and also significantly reduces a man's risk of contracting herpes, syphilis, or HIV during unprotected intercourse. Many men and women also like the appearance of an exposed glans.

On the other hand, opponents of circumcision argue that the foreskin protects the glans and lubricates it, thus supporting its ability to glide. Many people wonder why give up the foreskin if you don't have to?

Whether circumcised or uncircumcised men experience more arousal is a question for which there are no clear answers. There are men who claim an uncircumcised penis is more sensitive—and others who claim the opposite. Some women feel that the broad rim that is formed when the foreskin contracts behind the glans is stimulating during intercourse, and indeed there are penis rings available for the glans for this reason. (These are not to be confused with potency rings, which are applied at the base of the penis, not across the glans.)

Many doctors suggest circumcision to men with constricted foreskins (a condition that occurs in about one in ten men), as an alternative to encountering pain during intercourse or having to pull back the foreskin by hand. Whether circumcised or not, it is important is to accept the lingam as it is. Remember that however it is, it is wanted and wonderful.

▲ Massaging the Glans

1. Create a comfortable, relaxing space. You may wish to include nice music, candles, and a few essential oils. Prepare for the massage of the glans by touching the body first, or begin with a full-body massage as described on page 127.
2. Lovingly apply oil to the entire lingam and massage the shaft. Once a pleasant arousal has built up, gently and carefully pull back the foreskin if there is one, and touch the spot under the glans on the bottom of the lingam (meaning the side of the shaft that in the non-erect

lingam faces the testicles; if the lingam is resting against the stomach, this side of the shaft is facing up). This is where the frenulum is, with its very sensitive nerve endings. Gently massage this area by making circular movements with your thumb and using plenty of lubricant. The other hand can play with the nipples or gently stroke the body. If you're receiving this massage, note your sensations, be present, and take deep breaths.

3. Using both thumbs, massage the areas to the left and the right of the frenulum by stroking up and down; this is one of a man's most sensitive areas. A nice variant is to rub the skin of the frenulum between your thumb and index finger.

4. Now place your hand like a hat above the glans and massage the lingam in the hollow of your palm by moving it forward and back. For most men this creates an entirely new, fantastic feeling of arousal. When receiving this massage, try to enjoy the feelings that arise; breathe deeply and give in to spontaneous movements of your body. Let your partner know if you are getting close to orgasm; in this case he or she should remove hands from the lingam, but continue stroking the rest of your body.

5. Massage the glans by moving your fingers from top to bottom in a turning motion, as if squeezing lemons. A variant of this is to slide the fingers back and forth along the back edge of the glans. At this point, the recipient may be ready to finish with an orgasm.

The Lingam Root

The actual beginning of the lingam—the root—stretches about seven centimeters into the pelvis. It is located directly above your pubococcygeus (PC) muscle, and can be easily felt on your perineum. As noted above, the lingam root forms the back end of the urethra spongy body, which branches out like an onion.

When a man becomes sexually aroused, the root swells and emerges like an elongated bump from the perineum, which is why it is also called the "hidden penis." Below the lingam hill it emerges from the body into the shaft, ending in the glans (see figure 1.3 on page 12).

It is very rewarding to get in touch with one's root, since this area connects you to your first chakra—the foundational strength and joy of life. Remember that without roots, there are no flowers. From the root you can direct sexual energy into the glans, noticeably strengthening its flow.

The Reflex Zones of the Lingam

Many men rush through masturbation, trying to attain a quick erection and ejaculation by focusing on familiar techniques. For quick pleasure and to release sexual tension, there is nothing wrong with this. But from the Taoist perspective, the lingam has reflex zones—just like the ears or the feet—and they should all be stimulated from time to time.

The table below shows how each region of the lingam is connected to specific organs, feelings, etc. To find the individual regions, divide the lingam shaft (excluding the glans) into three parts. The first lingam ring is at the spot where the lingam exits the body, the second lingam ring corresponds to the middle of the shaft, and the third lingam ring is just before the glans.

You may wonder how it is possible to massage only one lingam ring, but in fact it's quite simple. Use one hand to lift the lingam. Place the thumb and index finger of your other hand on the lingam at the level you want to massage. Apply light pressure, and gently twist the lingam back and forth. In Chinese, this massage technique is called the "rope burn massage." The following information reflects the teachings of Taoism but has not been confirmed scientifically. You can explore it and try what is relevant for you.

Let's begin with the first ring. At the lower third, where the lingam shaft exits the body, you will find the reflex zone for the kidneys. If you want to stimulate the energy of your kidneys (your Water element), then massage this area lovingly, perhaps with a little lotion or oil. By stimulating the kidney zone you can help to resolve feelings of fear or unfulfilled longing. You can also develop your creative potential and learn to like being where you are.

The ring around the second third of the lingam shaft corresponds to your liver and the Wood element. Massage of this area can help to reduce feelings of anger, and replace them with joy and effective action.

Massaging the final third of the shaft will stimulate the spleen and pancreas. These correspond to the Earth element and will alleviate worries. Stimulation of this zone can also help with a lack of self-confidence or oversensitivity to outside criticism.

By gently massaging the sides of the glans (using lotion or oil), you will stimulate the lungs and your Metal element. This will help you to understand your needs and to take responsibility for your life.

In the middle of the glans are the reflex zones for the heart, which are sufficiently stimulated in any lingam massage.

The tip and bottom of the glans are connected to the pituitary gland, the pineal gland, the prostate, the adrenal glands, and the thymus. It is possible to stimulate these glands in a pleasant way during lingam massage, but the massage has to be approached very carefully to find the best level of stimulation.

▲ Lingam Self-Massage
for the Prostate

Massage the glans of your lingam by taking it between your index and middle fingers and using your thumb to gently press its tip. This gently stimulates the prostate gland, with positive effects on your libido. This massage also helps to prevent prostate problems. Remain attentive during this exercise—if you feel the need to ejaculate, pause and tense your PC muscle. In Chinese, this exercise is called "rubbing the turtle head."

According to Taoist teaching it is good for the organism as a whole to simply hold the lingam like a stick, something that many men automatically do unconsciously while falling asleep.

TAOIST REFLEX ZONE CORRESPONDENCES OF THE LINGAM

Region	1st lingam ring	2nd lingam ring	3rd lingam ring	Sides of the glans	Tip of the glans
Organ	Kidney	Liver	Pancreas	Lungs	Heart
Element	Water	Wood	Earth	Metal	Fire
Negative quality	Fear	Anger	Worry	Rage	Impatience
Topic	Unfulfilled desire	I am ignored	I'm not good enough	Nothing is allowed	I am shocked
Unresolved	Dishonesty	Meddling	Insecurity	Lack of intimacy	Mistrustful
Strength	Stamina	Joy of life	Stability	Structure	Internal purity
Path	Creativity	Vitality	Harmony	Concentration	Regeneration
Resolved	Pioneer	Optimist	Diplomat	Specialist	Philosopher
Scent	Ylang ylang	Sandalwood	Jasmine	Rose	Chamomile

The Perineum and the "Point of a Million Pieces of Gold"

The perineum is a very important area for your sexuality. It is located between the scrotum and the anus, and as mentioned above, is a place from which the "hidden penis" can be felt and massaged. Also on the perineum, directly across from the anus, is the so-called point of a million pieces of gold, known as the *jen mo* point among Taoists. If you feel that you are about to ejaculate and want to delay your orgasm, you can press this soft point right behind your penis base gently but surely. You will notice that you can press your finger in as far as the second joint.

Taoist teaching explains that pressure on this point causes energy to rise through the meridians—the body's energy pathways, which originate here—instead of leaving the body as it would during ejaculation. Applying pressure on the *jen mo* point just before (not during) climax cuts off the spermatic duct from the urethra, thereby reducing the pressure to ejaculate. This requires a bit of practice as it is not easy to locate the spot precisely enough to close the spermatic duct completely, but it does result in additional time for the massage. If an ejaculation is already in process, pressure on the *jen mo* point will prevent the excretion of sperm, causing you to ejaculate internally. This means the semen will be diverted into the bladder and excreted with the urine, causing it to appear slightly milky.

Despite these possibilities, the deeper pleasures of exploring this area are less about controlling ejaculation and more about enjoying the sensations. Directly behind the perineum is the prostate, which can generate feelings of great pleasure. Massage it from the perineum when you are already pleasantly aroused, since your body is geared to build pleasure from the front to the back. At this point, pressure on the prostate via the perineum will increase the blood flow to your penis, causing it to pulsate pleasantly.

The Prostate

The prostate is a male gonad that produces the majority of seminal fluid, which forms ejaculate in combination with semen cells from the testicles, the secretions of the seminal vesicles, and the secretions of the Cowper's or bulbourethral glands. The secretions from the prostate are milky and slightly sour, giving spermatic fluid its characteristic smell. They also contain many enzymes needed for fertilization. Mainly, the secretions from the prostate give the sperm mobility.

In the body, the prostate is located below the bladder. It looks something like a heart-shaped chestnut, which at its base is connected to the base of the bladder.

Unlike the lingam, the prostate is not visible from the outside and

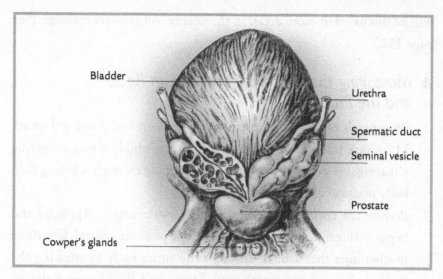

Bladder

Urethra

Spermatic duct

Seminal vesicle

Prostate

Cowper's glands

Fig. 1.7. Location and shape of the prostate

remains a largely unexplored erogenous zone. While your prostate can be massaged to some degree via the perineum, the most direct way to reach it is through your anus.

The prostate is surrounded by elastic connective tissue and is composed of two side lobes and a middle lobe. Within these lobes are dozens of individual glands, surrounded by smooth muscle strands. The muscle strands contract during ejaculation, propelling prostatic secretions into the urethra. At the same time, sperm are released from the seminal vesicles into this portion of the urethra.

For a man who is not aroused, having his prostate touched is generally rather unpleasant. But after a certain level of arousal, massage of the prostate can be quite pleasurable and can even lead to orgasms—much like the G-spot for women. Orgasms from the prostate are very different from those caused by stimulating the penis. They tend to connect men with their receptive sides, causing pleasure to spread more deeply and broadly throughout the body.

The back of the prostate touches the rectum, which is why it can be explored and stimulated with the fingers through the anus, which will be discussed in more detail in the chapter on prostate massage. (See page 158.)

▲ Massaging the Perineum, the Lingam Root, and the Prostate

1. By yourself or with a partner, find a pleasant and protected room. Make sure that your body (or your partner's body if you are giving a massage) is properly prepared, for example through a loving full-body massage or tender, gentle stroking.

2. Prepare the entire lingam by sensually awakening it. Apply oil and begin with gentle stimulation to create a pleasant arousal. Continue to distribute that arousal through the entire body by stroking the limbs, belly, and chest with your hands, and then begin exploring the perineum—the area between the testicles and anus.

3. Feel the bump below the testicles that is formed by the root of the lingam. Massage this area thoroughly by stroking repeatedly with your hands or thumb from the anus toward the testicles or from the thighs toward the perineum. While doing this you can also use your thumb and fingers to touch the lingam root, rubbing and massaging it gently. Make sure to ask your partner how he would like to be touched, and give him space to communicate his emotions.

   As a recipient, how does this touch of your root feel? How strongly and intensely do you want to be touched at this spot? Do you feel a gentle pulsating or swelling of the lingam root? If so, take this in, breathe, and continue to relax. Perhaps the feelings are unpleasant, since the perineum is often a neglected area, and thus is often tense or blocked. If this is so, breathe deeply into the painful feelings, which may help to resolve them. If the pain is too strong, stop the massage and ask your partner to simply rest his or her hand on your perineum. Feel the warmth and the energy that flows from the hand into the your body. Relax and be fully present—do not be discouraged, as even in the next massage, the pain may be much less.

4. If you would like to continue at this point, trace the lingam root

back toward the anus. Pay attention to the spot where your fingers come upon a soft area into which you can press deeply—the *jen mo* point. Behind it is the prostate. Massage this area carefully but thoroughly with two or three fingers. The prostate will feel like a small, solid, round rubber ball. If you are giving the massage to a partner, ask your partner whether this is the right spot, and continue to get feedback from him. You will probably notice that you can press quite strongly in this soft area. You can also carry out a vibration massage by pressing your fingers lightly onto the prostate and gently vibrating them. While doing this, vary your speed and pressure to make sure the experience is pleasant for your partner. Do not be discouraged if he does not feel much initially; this is an area that has to be thoroughly explored before it begins—probably very soon—to give back pleasure and deep emotions.

5. While exploring the perineum, continue to use one hand to stimulate the lingam. You can massage both areas simultaneously, and then one after the other. Pay attention to whether the awakening of the root causes the lingam to respond differently. If so, how? Play with this and continue to increase arousal as far as possible while remaining relaxed and pleasant.

6. Once you are close to ejaculation, press your middle finger gently but firmly into the *jen mo* point. (If you are giving the massage to a partner, ask him where exactly this point is, and press into it.) Take deep breaths, visualizing with each inhalation the energy rising from your perineum along your spine, and flowing down the front of your body back into the perineum as you exhale. What is happening inside your body at this moment? Do you feel the energy spreading through your cells? Remain fully present. Perhaps you will feel the pressure on the *jen mo* point stopping your ejaculation reflex; on the other hand, your need to ejaculate may increase. Whatever the case may be, try to fully enjoy what is happening. If you want, make sounds, move your pelvis around; breathe in and out through your mouth while moaning loudly.

7. You can repeat this exercise two to three times, if it is possible to do so easily while remaining relaxed. Each time, continue to a point just before you ejaculate. Can you begin to feel how—even without ejaculating—a feeling of orgasm is spreading through your body? Enjoy this wavelike spread of energy. If you don't feel it, don't be disappointed; try instead to and honor whatever you *do* feel. Take your time and enjoy the journey.

Scrotum, Testicles, and Epididymis

The scrotum is a loose-hanging bag of skin that is soft and movable. It has large pores and is slightly hairy. The scrotum is connected to the body between the lingam and the perineum and, as noted above, is comparable to the outer labia of women. The scrotum is surrounded by a thin layer of tissue, the *tunica vaginalis*.

Muscle cells within the scrotum allow it to grow large in heat and to tighten in cold and during sexual arousal. The two oval testicles in the scrotum move upward when the scrotum contracts. Fear and shock also lead to a contraction of the scrotum, causing the testicles to become small and pull tightly against the body.

Each testicle is connected to the scrotum by a spermatic cord, which consists of muscles, fascia, blood vessels, a spermatic duct, and nerves. Although the testicles can be felt from the outside, they are part of the internal reproductive organs, just like the epididymides, spermatic ducts, seminal vesicles, Cowper's glands, and prostate. As such, your "crown jewels," "nuts," "kiwis," or "balls of fire" will enjoy a gentle touch like the glans, perineum, and prostate.

Up until the late sixteenth century, testicles were more important symbols of masculinity and creative potential than the lingam. In biblical times, our ancestors held a hand above their testicles when taking an oath to affirm their honesty. Indeed, the word *testicle* comes from Latin and means "witness." The root of the word survives in terms such as *testimony* and *testament*.

The testicles are the male gonad and thus analogous to the female

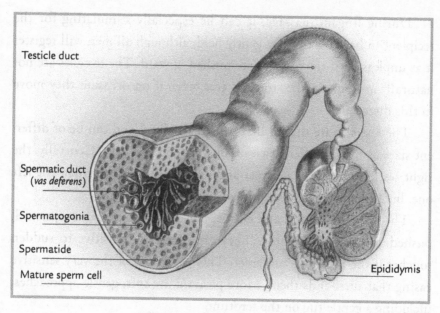

Testicle duct

Spermatic duct
(*vas deferens*)

Spermatogonia

Spermatide

Mature sperm cell

Epididymis

Fig. 1.8. Sperm production

ovaries. The testicles produce sperm, and in notable quantities: a man can produce up to 12 billion sperm cells over the course of his lifetime. Each sperm cell needs about 72 days to mature, a process that is controlled through hormones.

Sperm require a very particular temperature to mature, which is lower than normal body temperature. The scrotum, hanging loosely away from the body, provides an environment with an ideal temperature for sperm production and storage. Too much heat—for example from taking hot baths, wearing tight underwear, or heated seats in cars—lowers sperm production and should be avoided by men who wish to have children.

The testicles are composed of about 250 pockets divided by connective tissue. Each pocket is composed of thousands of winding testicle ducts, which produce spermatides, out of which the final semen cells grow. The blood supply of the testicles comes from the testicle artery (*A. testicularis*), which runs along the edge of the epididymis toward the so-called tail end of the testicles.

During lingam massage, it can be especially stimulating for the recipient to have his testicles gently held, although all men will register it as unpleasant if the testicles are pushed upward. The testicles are not naturally at home in the stomach area, even if on occasion they move in this direction.

The testicles are shaped like two small plums and can be of different sizes or rest at different elevations in the same man. Generally, the right testicle is somewhat larger and hangs a little higher than the left one, but there are many exceptions.

The testicles feel full and elastic, but do not enjoy being squeezed, pushed, or handled roughly. They are especially sensitive to sudden touches if the lingam is not erect. This is because of the very sensitive casing that surrounds them. More pleasant are soft, gentle approaches, including a gentle tug on the scrotum.

The testicles produce both sperm and the male hormone testosterone. While the hormones are absorbed by the body, the sperm moves to the epididymides, where they mature and are stored until ejaculation or reabsorption. The two epididymides look like small dragon tails. They are located on the back of the testicles and can be felt at the bottom of the scrotum. They are very sensitive to pressure and should be touched only very carefully during lingam massage. An experienced man can show his partner where each epididymis is located.

Spermatic Duct and Seminal Vesicles

The spermatic duct (*vas deferens* or *ductus deferens*) connects the epididymis with the urethra. It consists of layers of muscles and connective tissue. The seminal vesicles are located behind the bladder and end in the urethra. They produce fructose and prostaglandins, which together make up a large part of the content of ejaculate.

The ejaculate of a healthy man contains up to six hundred million sperm. Interestingly, however, only about 0.25 percent of these sperm are actually suitable for fertilization; the other 99.75 percent appear to have entirely different functions. This fact remained unknown for a long time, and it caused a sensation when Robin Baker asserted in his book *Sperm Wars* that the largest proportion of male sperm served to kill or block the sperm of other males.[3] An average ejaculation therefore contains only about one million potential "fertilization" sperm, along with about 300 million "killer" sperm and about 100 million "blocking" sperm.

The background to these sperm wars is a battle of the sexes. While the question of maternity is always clear, a man has to wonder whether he is truly the father of any particular child. A study of 500 people showed that women, especially during the fertile parts of their cycles, were more interested in affairs than men.[4] Scientists believe that the reason for this is a biological desire among women to take in different sperm samples to increase the probability of having the best genes for an eventual child. Men, on the other hand, want their own sperm to succeed—an undertaking assisted by the killing and blocking sperm cells, which are focused on eliminating "competitors."

As such, while the 0.25 percent of fertilizing sperm begin their odyssey to the egg, millions of killer and blocking sperm cells die off, as a way of blocking or destroying foreign sperm cells. For this, the killing sperm cells have a very strong fructose engine that allows them to quickly enter the cervix. DNA sensors help them to identify foreign sperm cells, which are then destroyed by toxins. The blocking sperm are more like kamikaze warriors and serve as a rear guard, forming a tough barrier that latches onto the walls of the vagina and blocks further access to the uterus, in case the woman sleeps with another man later on.

Interestingly, a man's older sperm cells will voluntarily sacrifice themselves for fresher cells. If the sperm of different men mix in a vagina, the ensuing battle over access to the egg cell can last days, resulting in only the healthiest and fittest sperm reaching the fertilization zones of the fallopian tube.

Whether fertilization actually takes place at this point depends largely on the woman, since it is she who unconsciously determines how long the sperm can stay in her body. If she decides against the male sperm, most of the ejaculate will flow out of her within thirty minutes, with the remainder being destroyed by her white blood cells. If, however, the woman or her yoni like the man, her body will allow the sperm to rest for up to five days in the "resting spaces" of the yoni. As soon as the egg is mature, the waiting sperm have their chance.

This, however, still does not ensure fertilization. To prevent weak sperm cells from fertilizing an egg, the female body has developed an elaborate obstacle course that can only be conquered by the strongest sperm. The fertilizing sperm cells have to cross zones in which the female body has hidden dangerous toxins, and have to overcome disorientating strategies, finding their way through labyrinths of dead ends in which they can die before finding their way back. This tests not only male strength, but also intelligence.

If some fertilizing sperm cells finally manage to reach the ripe egg, the most exhausting part of the journey is still ahead of them. The egg cell—huge compared to the tiny sperm—is protected by three layers. Thousands of sperm cells will surround the egg cell and attempt to penetrate its shell. Interestingly, it is not the fastest among them that wins this contest, but the most attractive one! The sperm that fits best with the egg cell is granted entry: the shell opens briefly to admit the single sperm cell and then closes again. All other sperm cells remain behind and die off. This process is very aptly described in medical terms as the "preconception attraction complex."

If it does happen that too many sperm cells enter the egg, the selection process was too mild, and the egg cell is killed by the toxins of the killer sperm.

▲ Massaging and Touching the Testicles

By yourself or with a partner find a pleasant room in which you will not be disturbed. Prepare the body for the following exercise with either a full-body massage or with gentle strokes across the whole body.

1. Begin by gently applying oil to the lingam, then stroking and stimulating it to create a pleasant erection. Then stroke your fingers along

the testicles and spermatic cords. Carefully touch the scrotum and feel the two testicles. How large are they and how do they feel between your fingers? Are there differences between the left and the right testicle?

2. Now take the spermatic cords between your fingers. Tug at the skin of the scrotum and massage it extensively. How does the touch feel for you (or for your partner, if you are giving the massage to someone else)? Is it pleasant or unpleasant? What is happening to your erection?

3. Now take the scrotum into your right hand, surrounding it until your hand is full. You can use your left hand to gently stroke the testicles—making circling movements, scratching them lightly, touching them with your fingertips, or massaging them with the ball of your hand. Some men will experience great pleasure during this exercise, while others might find it unpleasant. When giving this massage to a partner, pay attention to his face to make sure you register how this feels for him. If you are receiving this massage, continue to focus your attention on your testicles. How does the massage feel? How strongly or softly do you want to be touched here? Tell your partner exactly what is pleasant and arousing for you while he or she is carrying out this exercise.

4. Now use one hand to gently stimulate the lingam while the other lightly scratches the scrotum. If possible without pressure or tension, allow your arousal to rise up to a point just before ejaculation, then slow down or stop the touch and move the built-up energy throughout your body with gentle strokes. Breathe deeply into your pelvis and feel the energy in your entire body. Where exactly can you feel it?

5. If you want to, and if it can be done without stress, you can finish now with an ejaculation or by practicing the Big Draw (see page 109). Allow yourself enough time to recover afterward. If you have given the massage to a partner, speak with him about his experience.

The PC Muscle

The PC muscle plays a central role in increasing sexual energy and arousal in men. The muscle runs from the pubic bone to the coccyx and connects the anus and genitals with the buttocks and legs. It broadens like a butterfly throughout the pelvic floor, surrounding the prostate and controlling the opening and closing of the urethra, semen canal, and anus. If you need to urinate urgently and do not see a toilet anywhere, this is the muscle you have to rely on to keep your urine in. You can also feel it very noticeably if you try to press out every last drop while urinating.

The conscious strengthening of your PC muscle can lead to more enjoyable orgasms and stronger erections. In addition, men can use the PC muscle to separate their orgasms from ejaculation, because this muscle plays such a central role in controlling ejaculation. Finally, this muscle can be used to "body build" your lingam—focused training can strengthen and energize the penis. Good muscle tone can thus deliver power in love and life.

Think of your PC muscle as a drum. If a drum is too tight, its sound will be light and shrill, lacking depth and bouncing off the walls like a ball. On the other hand, if the drum is too loose, its sound will be absorbed—no vibration can build up, and the sound does not develop. But if the drum has good tension, the sound will develop in waves of depth and breadth, spreading outward. If you listen to this kind of drumming for long enough, the vibrations of the sound can cause you to enter a trance.

It is the same with your PC muscle. If the muscle is too tense and under constant stress, it won't develop feelings or sexual arousal. Your pelvis then becomes like a wall off of which all feelings bounce. On the other hand, if the PC muscle is too weak and has little or no tension, its energy is absorbed, and no feeling or sexual arousal can be maintained or expanded. You can't hold your urine, or control your erections, or strengthen your lingam.

Thankfully, you can strengthen your PC muscle and create good tension with a couple of simple exercises. These will allow your pelvis to build up sexual energy, as well as to expand and store it. As noted above, this can help strengthen your erections, and will allow you stronger, more intense orgasms, even enabling you to separate them from ejaculation. Focused training of the pelvic floor gives 80 percent of men with a weak penile spongy body an improvement in their ability to build and maintain an erection.

As with many exercises, breathing plays a central role in strengthening the pelvic floor. Deep breathing allows fresh energy and increased blood circulation to flow into the lingam, the pelvis, and the pelvic organs. If the muscles of the stomach, pelvic floor, and diaphragm cooperate during conscious inhalation and exhalation, the internal organs experience a wonderful strengthening massage.

When you inhale, your diaphragm lowers to make room for the expanding lungs. The stomach organs move forward, causing the pelvic floor to stretch and its muscles to relax. During exhalation, the diaphragm moves upward and presses against the lungs to support the out-breath. At the same time, the muscles of the pelvic floor contract inward and upward.

In men, contraction of the PC muscle stimulates the prostate. This triggers the release of hormones and endorphins that can improve mood and boost sexual vitality. So let's begin the sexercises.

▲ Exercise for the Muscles of the Pelvic Floor

Since the muscles of the pelvic floor are connected to one another, it is not possible to move the individual muscles in complete isolation from one another. However, it is possible and useful to differentiate them, and to use this as an effective training for the different groups of muscles. In the beginning, differentiating these groups of muscles may be difficult, but it will become easier with experience. For this reason, it is important to begin this exercise very slowly and with full alertness. Make sure that your stomach is relaxed during the exercises. After a few weeks of regular practice, you will be able to differentiate the muscles and to move them independently of each other.

1. Sit on a meditation cushion or on the front part of a chair, relaxed but straight. Place your feet parallel to each other on the floor. It is important to sit up straight for this exercise, so do not lean back.

2. Focus your attention on your pelvic floor. Then breathe in slowly, deeply, and with joy through your nose, and breathe out through your mouth, pushing your jaw forward as you exhale. Continue breathing in this way throughout the entire exercise.

3. **The gesture of the mare:** Breathe in deeply through your nose, then exhale through your mouth while contracting your rectal muscle. Relax the rectal muscle as you inhale again through your nose. Repeat this cycle of contraction and relaxation about thirty times: ten times very slowly, ten times at medium speed, and ten times quickly. Pause briefly after this exercise to feel its effects within your body.

4. **Kegel exercise:*** Again, breathe in through your nose and out through your mouth. As you exhale, contract your urethra as if you were trying to stop urinating in mid-stream. Relax while inhaling through your nose. Repeat this cycle about thirty times: ten times slowly, ten times at medium speed, and ten times quickly. Again, allow yourself a brief rest after the exercise to savor its effects.

5. **The Big Draw:** Breathe in through your nose, and while exhaling through your mouth, raise the middle of your pelvic floor, as if it were a hand making a fist. Relax this "fist" while inhaling through your nose. Repeat this exercise like the others—about thirty times: ten times slowly, ten times at medium speed, and ten times quickly, allowing yourself a brief rest afterward.

6. Inhale deeply and consciously through your nose. While exhaling through your slightly protruding jaw, contract your entire pelvic

---

*Named for Dr. Arnold Kegel, who systematized these ancient pelvic exercises and popularized them.

floor. Maintain this tension for six to ten seconds (with more experience, up to fifteen seconds). Then relax your pelvic floor while inhaling. Relax completely and take time to feel this relaxation. It is as important as the tension and should last at least as long. Repeat this exercise four to six times, or more if you wish.

7. Lie down on the floor, relax, and note the feeling of warmth in your pelvic floor. Feel how the energy spreads through your body and rejuvenates the cells.

You can discreetly train your PC muscle at any time: in your car while waiting for a traffic light to change, sitting in front of your computer, or brushing your teeth. Of course, you can also train it each time you urinate, by interrupting the urine stream six to eight times or even more often.

The conscious relaxation and contraction of your PC muscle, together with conscious breathing (relaxing during inhalation, contracting during exhalation) can also heighten your awareness during a lingam massage.

The Anus

The anal region brings us into contact with the innermost parts of a man and thus honors his "inner temple." There is no deeper way of touching a man. Opening himself to anal penetration enables a man to be in touch with his female characteristics of devotion, depth, and breadth.

The anal region is an erogenous zone with a high pleasure potential for men and women alike. However, because this area is the subject of many taboos in our society, it is often not well explored and even less sensually awakened. This is why it often goes untouched during lovemaking.

During childhood, most of us were told that we do not touch our orifices and definitely not to reach inside them because they are "dirty." Especially in the anal region, this leaves people with suppressed emotions, particularly in relation to topics such as control, power, and

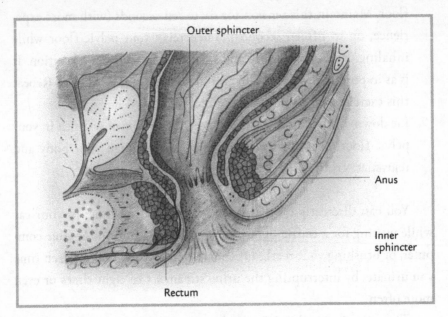

Fig. 1.9. The muscles of the anus

powerlessness. These suppressed emotions can manifest in chronic physical and emotional tensions.

We are also taught to judge our excretions. Stool is considered gross, stinky, and dirty. We generally don't want to look at or touch it. In general, we avoid getting in touch with the wet, processed products that leave our bodies.

But everything that flowers, smells sweet, and spreads its beauty will one day die, decompose, and return to dust. Everything that we enjoy putting into our mouths is processed in the stomach and intestines and excreted in part as stool through the anus. It is important that we are aware of this process and honor it, so that we can approach the anus sensually and without prejudices. Everything that our body can accept as nourishment is only available to use after the important work of the stomach and intestines is done. What is leftover is excreted so that it does not burden the body—just as a plant drops its flower when it has fulfilled its functions. Does this mean the flower should then be rejected?

The anal muscles are divided into the outer and inner sphincters.

The outer sphincter is controlled by the central nervous system and can, as explored above, be consciously contracted and relaxed. The inner sphincter, however, is controlled by the autonomous nervous system and can be consciously influenced only with extensive practice. The anus is about four centimeters deep and is surrounded by a calloused outer skin that is a little less sensitive than the other parts. But if we explore further inside, we reach the very sensitive mucous membrane of the intestines. Around the external skin of the anus—the anal rosette—are a large number of glands that give off a musky scent.

The anus is surrounded by a large number of nerve endings that are sensitive to the touch and are able to transport sensual and subtle feelings. Half (!) of all nerve endings of the pelvic area are located around the anus. Massaging the buttocks and perineum extensively before an anal massage leads to increased circulation and thus increased elasticity of the anus. Based on this knowledge, let us address some of the most common concerns and prejudices about anal massage:

Anal sex or anal massage means touching stool. This is only rarely the case, since the stool is collected in the large intestine, not the rectum. Neither penis nor finger penetrate to the large intestine. Nonetheless, it is useful to cleanse the anal canal before an anal or prostate massage, since in many people the intestines do not work exactly according to the textbooks. This does not require a complete enema, usually an anal douche will suffice. Nonetheless, as a rule of thumb, it is a good precaution that any fingers, penis, or dildo that have visited the anal region should be washed before further contact with the penis, vagina, or any kind of mucous membranes.

The sphincter will grow loose during anal sex or massage. This is not the case. At most, the sphincter may need some time to regulate itself after anal intercourse or anal massage, which in some cases can cause temporary flatulence.

Anal intercourse or massage causes hemorrhoids. This is not true. As long as the sphincter is not roughly stretched, and is carefully prepared with enough lubricant (petroleum jelly, bag balm, or other), an injury that could cause hemorrhoids is highly unlikely. However, those who suffer from hemorrhoids should forego anal intercourse or massage until the hemorrhoids have healed, since they might otherwise experience pain.

Penetration of the anal area should always happen very slowly. This is not correct either. The rectum is designed to excrete something out of the body rather than accept something in. That is why it reflexively contracts as soon as something wishes to enter. If we enter the anus too slowly, these contractions can range from unpleasant to painful. It is therefore recommended to spend plenty of time preparing the rosette, and then to insert the finger or penis gently but quickly.

To fully accept one's body requires being comfortable with all its ends and openings. A massage of the entire pelvic floor including the anal area supports the recipient in reclaiming constricted energies and bringing them into conscious experience. At first, new touch during anal massage can be painful—especially if there are physical or emotional tensions in the region. Therefore, the exploration of this inner channel should be a respectful process.

▲ The Anus Self-Love Ritual

Before exploring the anus, make sure that your fingernails are trimmed and that you don't have any rough spots on your middle or index fingers. It is useful to use Vaseline or Bag Balm for the exploration of this special area.

Begin by stimulating your penis; arousal accompanied by deep breathing and moaning facilitates letting go, and thus provides easier access to your inner sanctum.

1. Create a pleasant atmosphere in which you feel safe and comfortable. Stroke your whole body and begin with a loving massage of the lingam that includes your testicles and especially your perineum.

2. Turn onto your side, and massage the area around the anus with circling and touching movements. Be sure that your fingers are sufficiently lubricated. Pay attention to any sensations that arise during this massage. Does your touch vibrate throughout your body or does it stop somewhere?

3. Whenever you feel that the anal area has become fully relaxed, place one lubricated finger against the rosette, but do not penetrate the anus. Feel whether the rosette is attracting or repelling the finger. Breathe, and mentally observe the space between your finger and the rosette, and see what feelings rise up within you.

4. While keeping your finger on your anus, breathe deeply into it. Then feel into your finger. Imagine it growing longer and entering the anus. What does your finger feel? If your anus could talk or sing you a song, what would it say, what song would it sing?

5. Imagine that your anus is relaxed fully and that a finger of yours or a loved partner slides inside it easily. What emotions does this cause within you? Remain a few moments with these emotions.

6. Gently and lovingly massage the area around the anus. Carefully insert the lubricated finger into the anus when it is ready. Feel when your anus relaxes and contracts, and remain there for a moment until you have gotten used to the finger. Then try to consciously tense and relax the inner sphincter.*

7. Now explore your inner sanctum with love and a respectful presence.

8. The primary goal here is not sexual stimulation but conscious perception and physical relaxing of the anus muscles. Observe whether touching your anus has made you more sensitive, present, or emphatic. See chapter 4 for details of a more extensive anal and prostate massage.

THE SECRET OF THE ERECTION

There is a tribe in Africa that has an important annual ritual: on the longest day of the year, the entire village gathers and waits for its chief,

---

*For regular sphincter training, several products are available, including the Faktumat (available in two sizes in any pharmacy or through the internet), the "Ex Anal Angler" or the "G and P Stimulator" made by Orion, or a butt plug.

who then steps onto the veranda of his hut, lifts his loincloth, and displays his erection. On the day on which he can no longer display an erection, he is deposed from his position, since it appears that his days of fertility have passed.

However, the lingam represents more than physical fertility. It also represents creative potential, power, strength, and potency—and especially one's relationship to oneself.

Many men are likely to suffer from some form erectile dysfunction during their lives. Even though the absence of an erection may appear tragic at first, there are many ways of dealing with such an event positively. Even with a half-erect or non-erect penis you can visit a yoni, and receive a sensual and arousing lingam massage. It is more important to feel the lingam and be in loving touch with it than to have an erection. If you aren't aroused, the important thing is to admit and accept this fact. Don't interpret it as greed or rejection, need or abstinence—just accept it without judging it, and thus free yourself of tension and performance pressure.

Erections Are a Result of Relaxation

An erection cannot be forced—on the contrary, every man knows that any attempt to force an erection or even wish for one will only end in disaster. Men who are conditioned to solving problems through willpower are helplessly at the mercy of their lingams, which don't obey instructions. The more an erection is "demanded," the further into the distance it will recede. Fear and erections simply do not go together.

An erection requires both external stimulation and internal receptiveness. It is only when a man is relaxed and feeling comfortable with his partner that he can begin to feel sexually stimulated by touch, smell, his thoughts, or a look, massage, or caress. These impulses stimulate the nervous system and the erotic centers, causing the brain to release the hormones that the parasympathetic nervous system needs to become active.

The parasympathetic nervous system slows breathing and heartbeat and becomes active as we become quiet, amplifying our state of relaxation. When we are relaxed in this way, the "inflow arteries" of the lingam are able to open, releasing blood into the erectile tissue. This increased blood flow also exerts pressure on the veins in the lingam, virtually closing them off so blood does not flow out. This increases the volume of the erectile tissues by three to four times, and the lingam becomes erect. However, this wonderful event cannot be directed consciously; effort and struggle to attain it will usually achieve the opposite effect. It does happen during sleep, though: every 70 to 100 minutes, sleeping men get an erection, even without erotic dreams. It is part of the body's internal functioning to regularly supply the lingam with fresh oxygen—it's just a part of a healthy routine.

In the normal state, without sexual arousal, the sympathetic nervous system is active; it stimulates heartbeat and breathing, and causes the "inflow arteries" in the lingam to contract. With little blood, the lingam is flaccid and soft.

Stress and fear increase the activity of the sympathetic nervous system and cause the release of the stress hormone adrenaline—all events that withdraw blood from the lingam and distribute it to other parts of the body. As such, relaxation is an essential factor for a strong and lasting erection.

Relaxation, however, is something that feels very foreign to many men: from childhood onward, they are signaled that they are expected to perform on many levels. "You mean I don't have to work to get an erection?" is a common exclamation during a lingam massage.

Some time ago an older man came to the seminar and asked for a lingam massage. In the conversation beforehand he reported that he only rarely got an erection anymore, but that he wanted to experience an orgasm with ejaculation again. When we got to the lingam massage after an extensive, loving, and very relaxing full-body massage, he began moving his pelvis back and forth with great exertion, often holding his breath while doing this. His massage partner suggested that he try something completely new—perhaps moving his pelvis slowly and leisurely while saying to himself, "Feel, breathe, and enjoy—it is about joy. You can let go and give in to what you are feeling." As the man began to do this, it didn't take long for the desired erection to materialize, and for a very relaxed ejaculation to follow.

Supporting Erections

Any sexual problem is likely to cause insecurity in men, but nothing makes a man panic like the loss of his erection.

When a man feels that he can show himself as he is, and that he will find acceptance whatever happens, chances are that the psychological issues connected to his erectile dysfunction will resolve themselves. There are, of course, men who will still have problems achieving or maintaining erections, either for physical reasons, age-related reasons, or for reasons that remain unknown.

In the final analysis, however, there is no reason why a couple should not be able to enjoy each other with love and desire. The goal is not an erection, but mutual enjoyment; in this case, the ways of giving pleasure to your partner are unlimited and don't require an erection. Yoni and lingam massages can be an incredible gift in this regard. In addition, open conversation can be a step to a new, deeper level of intimacy.

Finally, it is important to remain playful with all of this; it is not about performance or points for effort. A person's sexuality is as unique as his or her fingerprints. Unexpected developments offer couples the opportunity to turn a burden into desire, frustration into enjoyment, and fear into openness. Where old trauma blocks the way, love and respect offer comfort and a way out. In this way impotence can be overcome, since "love heals all wounds."[5]

What Else Can You Do?

It helps to acknowledge that behind not being able to is often a not wanting to, usually unrecognized up to this point. Honoring this "not wanting" allows you to move on and ask what it is that you do want. Here a magical question can help: "If you woke up tomorrow and your sexual problem was magically resolved, by what feeling would you notice it, and how would you live?"*

Other emotional issues may be involved as well: ask yourself if you accept your partner just as he or she is, not necessarily as you think they should be. Is there more that you and your partner can be doing to help each other leave behind old gender roles and expectations? Are you able to recognize the depth of your natural sexual desires, as well as your partner's? Embark on a search together—sexuality can only work on a basis of equality.

PHYSICAL REASONS FOR ERECTION PROBLEMS

Until about thirty years ago, people thought that erection problems were exclusively a result of psychological causes. More recent research has shown that in 55 to 85 percent of cases, physical factors play a role in chronic erectile dysfunction.[6] These factors include:

▲ Arteriosclerosis. Certain lifestyle choices can worsen arteriosclerosis, including stress, lack of movement, excessive use of salt, and a diet high in trans fats.

▲ High blood pressure. If you have high blood pressure, you may be able to lower it by reducing your stress levels, changing your diet, and increasing your exercise. Medication will regulate blood pressure but may also have undesirable effects on your ability to achieve and maintain erections.

▲ Smoker's penis. Excessive smoking not only leads to a clogging of the penile arteries but also damages the sealing mechanism of the veins.

▲ Obesity.

---

*More information about magical questions like this one can be found in books about short-term therapy by Steve de Shazer.

- High cholesterol.
- Alcohol abuse. Overuse of alcohol can cause circulation problems as well as a degeneration of the *corpus mamillare* in the brain, which is responsible for our sexual behavior. It is well known that small quantities of alcohol can cause relaxation and reduce inhibitions, but once a person has drunk too much, nothing will happen down below.
- Blood flow problems in the perineum. Blood flow to the perineum can be adversely affected by stress, certain sports (such as cycling), or particular occupations. Sitting too much can also affect the circulation of the penis, as can underwear or pants that are too tight.
- Nervous system problems. The nervous system transmits sexual stimuli and ensures that certain enzymes are directed to the genital region. Surgery (especially on the prostate), injuries, neurological ailments, Parkinson's disease, and spinal problems (especially in the area of the sacrum) can all interfere with erectile function, as can nervous tension.
- Metabolism issues and diabetes. More than 50 percent of men suffering from diabetes will become impotent during the course of their lives; diabetes not only blocks the walls of blood vessels, but also damages nerves, preventing nerve impulses important for an erection from being transmitted.
- Hormone dysfunctions. Male sex hormones are formed in the Leydig cells of the testicles as well as in the adrenal glands. If not enough hormones are available to support erections, many men resort to aphrodisiacs or take PDE-5 inhibitors such as Viagra, which offer only temporary relief.

For a long time people thought that the formula for male arousal was very simple: more testosterone = more arousal, but today we know that this is not true. It has been discovered that a prehormone called dehydroepiandrosterone (or DHEA) contributes to sexual desire. DHEA is produced by the adrenal glands and is a precursor to other sexual hormones, including testosterone and estrogen.

▲ Excessive stimulation. The adrenal glands deal with both stress and arousal. Prolonged excessive stress on the adrenals—from overwork or even through overuse of hardcore pornography—can lead to erection problems. This can cause some men to need a continually stronger stimulus to become erect. The solution here is a gradual deprivation of stimulus to promote increased receptivity.

▲ Stress. Under the influence of stress hormones, the testicles reduce the production of testosterone. In both men and women, stress also leads to reduced production of DHEA. Stress is thus counterproductive for both erection and the ability to become aroused.

Focused Ways to Strengthen Erection Capacity

To promote good erections, we have to promote the flow of energy to the lingam. Any man, regardless of age, can promote the supply of oxygen to his lingam and maintain its elasticity through exercise. The following is a list of exercises that promote potency in men.

▲ Breath training: focused, relaxed inhalations into the pelvic floor, testicles, and penis.

▲ Sports and dance: skiing (stimulates circulation in the pelvis), tennis (stimulates ability to react to stimuli), salsa dancing (promotes circulation in the hip area), endurance sports.

▲ Strengthening of the pelvic floor: increases circulation in the pelvic area and thus increases the ability of the lingam to become erect.[7]

▲ Pelvic exercises: swinging, lifting, rocking the pelvis, as well as other motions.

▲ Body pump: exercise programs are very good for promoting circulation in the pelvic area. Classes are offered in many gyms.

▲ Chi machine: ten minutes a day promote the free flow of energy throughout the body.

▲ Feldenkrais exercises: promote deep relaxation and resolve stress on the cellular level. The "pelvic clock" exercise is particularly helpful for lingam health.

▲ Hot and warm footbaths: stimulate circulation.

▲ Muscle training: leg presses, abdominal training, and others.

▲ Inline skating: stimulates circulation in the pelvis.

▲ Trampoline jumping: about 15 minutes to strengthen the walls of blood vessels.

▲ Sexual body work.

▲ Yoga: exercises like the cobra not only promote circulation, but also improve body elasticity overall.

▲ Exercises from chapter two of this book—for example progressive muscle relaxation and breathing exercises.

▲ Exercise for Potency:
Lingam Self-Massage in the Bathtub

1. Fill the tub with warm water.
2. Enter the bath, then massage your lingam until it becomes big and erect. Remain aware while doing this: don't push yourself too quickly or suppress your reactions.
3. While continuing to massage your lingam with one hand, form a testicle ring with the index finger and thumb of your other hand. Pull your testicles slightly downward, but make sure not to ejaculate.

The warmth and pressure of the water stimulate both hormone production and blood circulation. More circulation also always means more feeling! After several days of practicing this exercise, you will observe that your erections have improved noticeably.

EJACULATION

At some point during puberty every boy experiences it: a sweet feeling accompanied by the excretion of a milky liquid from the lingam. For some, the first ejaculation comes as a complete surprise, sometimes even as a nocturnal emission—without any touch to the lingam at all. Over the following weeks, growing boys will then discover the marvelous sensations that can be caused by the rubbing, stroking, and touching of the lingam.

Unfortunately, today's youth are not taught how to masturbate lovingly. It thus becomes for them simply a way to resolve any kind of tension. Without understanding that his seed is a treasure, a young man does not learn to consciously connect masturbation with the act of loving himself; he doesn't learn to orient his love life toward sensual fulfillment.

Since young people normally receive only limited (if any) introduction to their sexuality—and these rarely provided lovingly—they often look elsewhere for sexual stimulation. Thus they might focus on the Internet, rather than learning to connect their own fantasies with the natural desire to touch themselves. All of these circumstances can make a natural and conscious approach to sexuality and ejaculation more difficult, which may be one reason why an increasing number of men suffer from premature ejaculation problems. To enable men to once again learn how to delay their arousal, how to expand and deepen their sensuality, requires bringing consciousness, slowness, acceptance, and joy into sexuality.

The Biology of Ejaculation

Although erections can begin in infancy, ejaculation is possibly only after puberty. As discussed on page 31, sperm are produced in the testicles and travel via the spermatic duct (or vas deferens) into the canal system of the epididymis, where they mature.

Ejaculation (from the Latin word for squirting or throwing) is triggered by the sexual center in the interbrain. At the same time, it uses receptors to stimulate the muscles of the bladder, causing it to close. This prevents the flow of sperm into the bladder and a mixing of sperm and urine. The nerve impulses from the sexual center of the interbrain have effects on the sympathetic nerve cells in the loin area of the spinal cord (the ejaculation center), which causes contractions in the genital channels, the spermatic ducts, seminal vesicles, and prostate.

An ejaculation consists of two parts: semen emission and ejaculation. During semen emission, the semen is propelled from the epididymis, the seminal vesicle, and the prostate into the posterior part of the urethra, where it mixes with the secretions of the gonads.

During the actual ejaculation, semen is moved forward in intervals and then fiercely ejected from the urethra at speeds of up to 40 kilometers per hour. This is achieved through rhythmic and coordinated contractions of the walls of the channels of the epididymis, the spermatic duct, the seminal vesicle, the prostate, and the urethra.

The Refractory Period following Ejaculation

After ejaculation, the refractory period follows. The lingam loses its erection as the sympathetic nervous system opens the venous backflow valves and blood flows out of the erectile tissues. The entire body slowly returns to its normal state. The swelling of the testicles is reduced, and they are lowered back into their original position. Muscles relax and breathing, pulse, and blood pressure return to normal. At this point, the glans is especially sensitive and any stimulation of it is perceived by most men as very unpleasant.

In general, most men are unreceptive to sexual stimulation immediately after ejaculation and prefer to be held. They experience an intense need for rest and sleep, giving the body the chance to recover. The reason for this abrupt decline in sexual interest after ejaculation is the release of prolactin—a hormone that acts as a "lust killer" and prevents the lingam from filling with blood and becoming erect. After a break—shorter among younger men—men will be ready to resume their sexual adventures.

In the time following ejaculation the male body makes concerted efforts to restore its semen. For this, the glands that are part of this process require raw materials, which are found in the blood. Blood draws these substances from food, or, if they are not immediately present there, from the liver, kidneys, spleen, or brain. A young man won't even notice the energy required for this process, although men in their later years often experience a slight weakening or fatigue after ejaculation—which can sometimes last for hours, although it will pass over the course of the day.

To counteract this feeling, it is helpful for older men to ingest natural vitamins and minerals—especially zinc—after ejaculating. A mixture of honey, propolis, and bee pollen has proven very useful, and can also be supplemented with royal jelly. It is this combination that is often used in mixtures that claim to increase potency or erections.

Some men experience a loss of energy after ejaculating, or even post-orgasmic depression, though they may be unaware of it. Post-orgasmic depressions can be prevented by consciously welcoming and enjoying orgasm, ejaculation, and the refraction period following it. Use this time to inwardly thank yourself and your partner for this beautiful feeling. Enjoy the relaxation, and know that your energies will automatically be restored by your body, even if it may take a little more time as you grow older. True love is among the deepest needs of every man and woman. I would be surprised to hear a man complain about a loss of energy that might occur after making love with a woman he loves; he knows that the melting wave-like dance that culminated in his flowing into her, came from love and devotion, and he would not begrudge the energy these require.

Sometimes an occasional ejaculation can be experienced as an energy gain, for example if a man has plenty of energy but has been feeling tense or overwhelmed. In this case, ejaculation may make a man feel revitalized. An energy gain can also occur if ejaculation was delayed by thirty to forty-five minutes during a lingam massage, followed by an intense orgasm with ejaculation. In these cases, men often tell me later that they continued to feel the experience for several days, as a feeling that strengthened them, because it brought them into touch with the "original" strength of their bodies.

For a man to be able to experience his sexuality with energy at any time, it is important that he to learn to separate orgasms from ejaculation, and to decide in sexual freedom whether or not to ejaculate. Because once ejaculation has begun, it should not be stopped. Thus it is important to be clear about what one wants when one approaches the point of no return. If you then decide to have an ejaculation, allow it wholeheartedly. This will give you more pleasure than a suppressed orgasm. It would be a shame to miss this wonderful feeling.

Repeated ejaculations in quick succession lead to greater feelings of fatigue, especially in older men. For this reason it makes sense for older men not to ejaculate as frequently. Instead, they can learn to separate orgasm from ejaculation, and thereby retain the strength and energy that are built up in the body after orgasm. If there is no ejaculation, this energy can then be distributed throughout the body to supports one's health, strength, and vitality.

In their youth, many men boast about being able to ejaculate several times in a row. But if a man learns to enjoy making love for longer before ejaculating, and to experience orgasms without ejaculation, he will possess a more enduring love power, which will enrich both him and his partners.

Premature Ejaculation (Ejaculatio Praecox)

Premature ejaculation refers to a man reaching orgasm more quickly than he or his partner wish. The ejaculation may come with little pleasure, and may also be accompanied by a disappointed partner, who may feel used and abandoned.

This problem is common among young, inexperienced men, but also occurs in men of all ages: they are aroused and want to visit the yoni, or the lingam massage has only just begun, and suddenly "it" happens, either before penetration or during the first movements in the yoni.

Ejaculation problems can be divided into genetic/predisposed and acquired ones, with the latter being far more common. Medically, premature ejaculation is defined as ejaculation after less than one minute in at least 50 percent of all attempts. Premature ejaculation was described by Latumann et al. in the "National Health and Social Life Survey" (NHSLS) as the most common of all sexual dysfunctions, occuring in 35 percent of men. The causes of premature ejaculation are unclear, although in many cases they are a result of psychological or acquired components.[8]

Premature Ejaculation—What to Do?

A lack of control over the ability to perform and enjoy sex is very disturbing for most men. This can lead to a vicious cycle in which the fear of premature ejaculation becomes a self-fulfilling prophecy. It is thus first of all important to accept the condition and accept yourself as you are, for example with the following affirmation: "Even though I ejaculate earlier than I want to, I accept myself completely!"

As always, relaxation is the first step to the solution. This allows you to accept consciously and without judgment what is happening in your body during sexual arousal—what feelings, emotions, and thoughts arise within you.

Premature ejaculation can have physical or mental causes. Physical causes include:

- ▲ Weakness of the muscles of the pelvic floor: almost all muscles that control ejaculation are linked directly or indirectly to the muscles of the pelvic floor. For this reason a focused PC muscle training can be very useful. See page 37 for a range of exercises designed to help strengthen the PC muscle.
- ▲ Infections in the prostate or urethra: this is rather rare, but can be diagnosed easily.
- ▲ Excessive arousal levels: for example through excessive consumption of coffee, taurine, meat, or chronic stress.
- ▲ Increased secretions of the sexual glands (semen blockage) or excess testosterone levels (more common among young men). In these cases it can be helpful to stimulate the lingam only minimally and

to consciously spread the energy throughout the body using long strokes.

As discussed above, erection and ejaculation are two reflexes that operate independently of each other. Thus an ejaculation can come from a flaccid or an erect lingam. An urge to ejaculate can exist even if the lingam is still small and flaccid. In this case it is important to ensure relaxation and to reduce the direct stimulation of the lingam.

Spiritual and Mental Causes

Stress in one's job or life, relationship problems, and an overall lack of harmony can be found among almost all men suffering from premature ejaculation. Anger, frustration, or unconscious rejection can also contribute to premature ejaculation; sometimes the body is expressing that something is wrong in the relationship.

Premature ejaculation can also be an escape from too much intimacy. Or it can come from a habit of masturbating quickly, perhaps due to feelings of shame or guilt. Finally, the impulse to quickly escape a sexual situation instead of fully enjoying it can often be a barrier to the conscious perception of sexuality.

Lingam massage offers a way to find a clear and feeling connection to your own sexuality. This is based on perceiving what is true, focusing on taking it slow, and on increasing the ability to derive joy. This allows you to feel whatever it is that you feel, and to remain fully present in the here and now. You relax in whatever it is that your body signals you.

Take the time to breathe deeply and consciously during lingam massage and note where exactly you are with your arousal on a scale of 1 to 100. One hundred is the point of no return, meaning that the ejaculation has now begun and can no longer be stopped. The more you are able to rate your arousal, the more consciously you can accompany the process.

The best suggestions for avoiding premature ejaculation are of little use if you continue to focus on small solutions, and give in to the pull of the ejaculation reflex, either from habit or an addiction to "relief." It is unequivocally a decision to approach the big solution and experience a truly deep level of sexual fulfillment that will help you learn to keep breathing, delay your ejaculation, and circulate the growing arousal throughout your entire body.

Many men report that an orgasm that occurs after only a few minutes is like a small spark compared to the imposing fires of orgasms that take place thirty to sixty minutes after a wave of sexual-erotic arousal throughout the body. The cosmic orgasms that are experienced by many during lingam massage often have strengthening and fulfilling effects that last for days. Once you have made the decision within yourself to attain this, the most important precondition for avoiding premature ejaculation has been met.

During a lingam massage, you can agree with your partner on a clear signal (for example lifting your hand), to be given as you approach the point of no return. Among people with less experience, it is important to give this signal at 70 or 80 percent. Among those with more experience it is sufficient to give the signal at 95 or even 98 percent. The stimulation is then stopped immediately, and the erotic energy distributed throughout the entire body with strokes. During these moments, deep breathing can relieve over-excitement—and eventually, premature ejaculation.

At the same time, you can contract your PC muscle and concentrate on moving the energy upward through your body, perhaps accompanied by a light shaking of your limbs. This causes a gradual reprogramming of your sexuality—you experience your sexuality consciously and thus with significantly more joy, and as a side effect develop more sexual maturity.

Decisive for this new experience is your presence in the here and now, whether you're experiencing lingam massage or lovemaking with your partner. Especially among men with premature ejaculation problems, drifting off into sexual fantasies can make control and consciousness impossible. That is why it is important to breathe consciously, which prevents a detour into fantasies.

Trying to impose your will on the situation will likely backfire. Premature ejaculation is not avoided through effort, but through consciousness, a clear decision, relaxation, and giving in.

Other Help

▲ Relaxation exercises: biofeedback training, meditation, the exercises described earlier in this chapter, and especially the progressive muscle relaxation exercise described in chapter 2.

▲ Visualization: every morning before getting out of bed, visualize yourself loving for a long time and with great enjoyment, and in control of your ejaculation. If necessary, use this visualization to prepare for the stop-and-go method described below.

▲ Training of the pelvic floor: this can prevent premature ejaculation caused by a weakness of the pelvic floor, which can often occur in old age.[9]

▲ Training of the PC muscle: contract the PC muscle if you feel the need to ejaculate. See page 37 for PC-training exercises. The Taoist master Mantak Chia also recommends clenching your teeth and rolling your eyes upward as you contract your PC muscle during urination. This may sound strange, but it works to strengthen the PC muscle.

▲ Pressing the "point of a million pieces of gold" (see page 25).

▲ Remain in the here and now: do not fantasize, do not think of someone or something else during stimulation, but stay present.

Complete Ejaculation Control

Complete ejaculation control depends on being able to separate ejaculation from orgasm. Neurophysiologically, orgasm and ejaculation are two completely different processes. Ejaculation itself does not cause the feeling of orgasm, but is simply a physical act that moves ejaculate out of the body. Orgasm is an intense energy experience that occurs—in men without training—fractions of a second before ejaculation.

Sexually experienced men have a good perception of their own arousal and are thus aware of their ejaculation point before it happens. Fulfilling sexuality for men means consciously accompanying one's own sexual energy.

The lingam self-massage, combined with the stop-and-go method described below, can help you get into touch with your own rhythms of ejaculation and orgasm; it can help you learn to separate these two events and experience energy with the Big Draw. At the same time, this self-love ritual is also useful if you simply want to learn how to delay and enjoy ejaculation.

▲ Lingam Self-Massage Combined with the Stop-and-Go Method

1. Before you focus on your genitals, remember to touch and massage the rest of your body, especially your stomach, thighs, and nipples.
2. Massage yourself as you like. Stimulate your entire lingam, testicles, and perineum.
3. Pay attention to your arousal curve. Try to trace the beginning of arousal: note the tingling of your lingam root, observe the stages of erection, observe the quickening of your breath and pulse.
4. Increase your stimulation until just before the critical point of no return, then stop, breathe calmly, and contract your PC muscle around your prostate. Beyond this you can delay ejaculation by now pressing on your *jen mo* point (see page 25), gently pulling your testicles downward, squeezing the tip of your lingam with your hand, or simply using your mind to visualize doing the same. The most important thing is to observe the stages of your arousal and stop at the right time—before ejaculation is triggered.
5. If you need fantasies to become aroused, imagine that your lingam is being received by a beautiful yoni, since this comes closest to the reality of sexual experience. But it's best to entirely avoid drifting into fantasies.
6. The key to this exercise is to listen and feel what is happening inside you, to breathe deeply into your pelvis, and to learn to consciously

feel your own sexual reactions. Observe closely where you are on an erection scale from 1 to 100.

7. If you are feeling very aroused, visualize your sexual energy flowing upward along your spine to the top of your head as you inhale, and back down along the front of your body to your perineum as you exhale. Allow your sexual energy to flow easily and spread throughout your body.

8. Repeat this stopping and starting several times until you feel more comfortable with it. Continue to stroke your entire body to distribute your energy, and continue touching your testicles and perineum. Can you feel your energy spread throughout your body in waves? Can you feel it circulating around?

9. If you like, you can reward yourself with an ejaculation after some time. But if you want to keep it back and use this energy instead for your self, for your health and creativity, or for a full body orgasm without energy loss, you should practice the Big Draw at this point (see the detailed description on page 109). Visualize this sexual energy being distributed throughout your body, being absorbed by all of your cells, and allow your body to vibrate or shake lightly. Enjoy your orgasm as you would any other and take your time to fully feel this feeling as it ebbs.

10. Once you feel reasonably comfortable with this exercise, ask your partner to stimulate your lingam. This is not about the precise techniques discussed later in the book, but about the awareness of both partners during stimulation. Give hand signals early on as you approach the point of no return and maintain control of your ejaculation to allow the energy to spread throughout your body.

11. When your partner stops the stimulation, breathe deeply. Ask your partner to use strokes to spread your sexual energy from your pelvis throughout your body.

12. If it feels right for both of you, and you want to, you can reward yourself with an ejaculation, a visualization of the spread of energy, or the Big Draw.

Let's conclude with two techniques that make it easier to move sexual energy upward along your spine using both visualization and breathing. The expansion of energy and consciousness that is accomplished through the delay or complete absence of ejaculation in favor of emphasizing more subtle internal experiences, is known in two variations: the Microcosmic Orbit and the Inner Flute.

The Microcosmic Orbit

The Microcosmic Orbit is the main energy channel in the body. It consists of the back and front channels, which in Chinese medicine are known as the Governor Vessel and the Conception Vessel. The back channel (Governor Vessel) runs from the tip of the coccyx along the spine up to the top of the head and then down the center of the face to the gums. The front channel (Conception Vessel) runs from the tip of the tongue along the midline of the front of the body down to the perineum. During lingam massage you can visualize and feel how the sexual energy moves upward along the Governor Vessel and then downward along the Conception Vessel. Taoist yoga sees in this practice the key to the healing of the body and a whole-body enjoyment of sexual energy.

The Inner Flute

Imagine a vertical line along your body that runs like an internal flute from your perineum to the top of your head. Along this line lie the endocrine glands that are responsible for the energy levels in your body. Using consciousness and breathing, you can let your sexual energy flow upward along this inner flute, carrying physical and spiritual vitality. If necessary, you can use chakra breathing exercises to cleanse the channel between your root chakra and your crown, making it easier for sexual energies to permeate. Those who have used this method report a good control over their ejaculations, combined with important spiritual experiences.

Preventing ejaculation and distributing sexual energy require some practice and may feel strange at first, but are well worth the effort. If

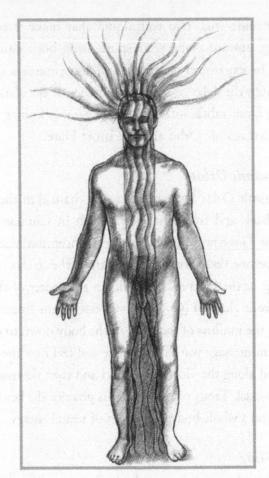

Fig. 1.10. The Inner Flute (from Margo Anand)

you feel that the sexual energy remains stuck in your body after the exercise, practice rhythmic breathing for another ten to thijrty minutes (which ensures a good distribution of energy), before relaxing for a few additional minutes.

The Inner Flute, breathing in the Microcosmic Orbit, and the Big Draw are described more extensively in chapter 2. You can continue to practice these exercises, which will further help you integrate your sexual experience. Over time, you will become more aware of the healing power of sexual energy as it spreads through your body, nourishing and maintaining it from the inside.

THE MALE ORGASM

Even before Wilhelm Reich coined the phrase "orgasmic potency," human beings knew how important orgasmic experiences are for all of us. The orgasm is an opportunity to feel one's own power and energy, as well as something larger than oneself. Many people discover new creativity from their orgasms, which then finds expression in other aspects of their lives. Above all, orgasms are healthy for all parts of our being: our physical, mental, and spiritual selves benefit from the increased well-being that orgasms provide, giving us the courage and joy to participate in life.

Recent studies from Bristol in the UK have shown that sexual intercourse at regular intervals lowers the risk of stroke by up to 50 percent. Moreover, men between the ages of 45 and 60 who joyfully and regularly celebrate their sexuality have a significantly higher life expectancy.[10]

There is almost no area of life in which orgasms would not have a healing effect. They are a sleeping aid and an anti-depressant, an anti-aging cure and a stress reducer—all due to the release of dopamine and the activation of the brain's pleasure center, the *nucleus accumbens*. Even pain can be alleviated by the endorphins released during orgasm, especially migraines and other headaches. The post-orgasm increase in blood-oxygen levels vitalizes the body's cells and organs while DHEA rejuvenates men physically, mentally, and spiritually.

Studies show that sexual repression makes men aggressive, destructive, and tyrannical, while men with fulfilling orgasms have something that they want to build and contribute to the beauty of the world. Andreas Krüger, the head of the Hanemann School in Berlin, emphasizes that "orgasmically lived sexuality makes people mild!" Thus it is not sex that is bad for health, but prohibitions against sex, or moral condemnations of it. Of course, if you are suffering from health problems, you should discuss any sexual activity with your doctor.

Multiple Orgasms

For many men, orgasm signifies the end of a sexual experience. But as we know by now, multiple orgasms are possible for conscious and creative men during a sexual encounter; they are not the exclusive domain of women. The key to multiple male orgasms is remembering that one does not always have to ejaculate to experience a satisfying orgasm.

▲ Riding the First Wave

1. Enjoy the stimulation and arousal during lingam massage or love-making.
2. Stop just before ejaculating, take a deep breath, avoid further stimulation, relax, and wait until your arousal decreases a bit. If necessary, clench your teeth, roll your eyes upward, or squeeze your glans between your fingers until the urge to ejaculate is reduced. (Try these methods to see whether they work for you, as they are different from man to man). Then begin anew.
3. Shortly before the point of no return, contract and release your PC muscle a few times to experience small or large storms and orgasmic waves, which may shake your body.
4. Gently tug at your "crown jewels" (testicles), or ask your partner to. If you pull them downward at the right time (using the ring grip), you can noticeably delay ejaculation. At the same time, this grip increases sexual receptiveness. Begin by practicing this a few times on your own.
5. Conclude this experience either with a strong ejaculation that lasts longer than two seconds, a Big Draw, or a distribution of energy through your entire body. Rest for some time afterward.

If you practice this exercise, it will allow you to ride the waves of ecstasy for hours on end. How long the so-called plateau phase lasts depends entirely on you and how capable you are of recognizing your arousal curve, and how long you want to prolong it. Up to a certain point, you can consciously direct the plateau phase, which will increase its effects throughout your body the longer it lasts.

The Role of Breathing and the Big Draw in Male Multiple Orgasms

Preventing ejaculation by itself does not cause a full-body orgasm. For this, it is important that you give in emotionally to what is happening, and use your breathing to heat up your sexual energy (see the section on breathing in chapter 2).

However, delaying ejaculation during lingam massage does increase your sexual energy minute by minute. When you get close to your point of no return, orgasmic energy begins to spread throughout your body, especially if your partner strokes your energy around while you breathe strongly and consciously. More and more strength builds up, and eventually floods the centers of light in your brain. At some point you will switch to a higher state of energy, paving the way to experience an intense, cosmic full-body orgasm.

A full-body orgasm goes deeper and lasts much longer than a regular one, which is often over within half a second. During a fully-body orgasm, the entire body fills with strength, heat, well-being, and shudders of joy. These feelings extend beyond the genital area and circulate everywhere. Afterward, you don't feel weakened or exhausted, but full of energy and activity as if you could go out and pick up trees.

The Big Draw (see page 109) offers another way to support the cosmic multiple orgasm. This technique will help you to distribute built-up energy throughout your body, using conscious contraction and relaxation of different muscles to create another energy rush. When combined with rhythmic breathing, the Big Draw also prevents the kinds of sexual blockages that can happen to inexperienced men when they don't ejaculate.

The Big Draw helps sexual energies to flow upward through the central channel—from the loins to the top of the spine. This exercise can create an incredible feeling of peace and happiness while also increasing energy.

Orgasm Consciousness during Lingam Massage

Lingam massage offers the opportunity to try out subtle variations in stimulation and broaden one's range of sexual experience. During lingam massage, men learn to consciously direct and accompany their orgasms, frequently increasing their sexual pleasure and leading to more intense climaxes. Awareness can be enhanced and encouraged by the massage giver, who can continue to spread energy throughout the body. During stimulation, tension and relaxation remain in balance with one another.

▲ Felt and Spoken Exercises during Lingam Massage

1. Ask your partner to give you a thorough lingam massage.
2. Try to be aware of all the qualities of the touch, take deep breaths, and remain fully present. Become your feeling.
3. Allow yourself to feel deep inside the emotions and sensations that arise during the massage. Remain in the here and now. Every once in a while, you can briefly relay these feelings to your partner, without judging or interpreting them. Continue to feel within yourself and perceive what comes up. Experience how one layer after another peels away. This process is amplified by the continued strokes across your body. Try maintaining eye contact with your partner, then closing your eyes; decide which feels better for you.
4. Observe your arousal curve. Try to trace the increases in your arousal levels: feel the tingling of your lingam root, observe the stages of your erection, note the quickening of your breathing and your pulse.
5. Continue to tell your partner exactly where you stand with your arousal.
6. Once you are at about 70 to 80 percent, give your partner a clear signal so that he or she can stop the stimulation and distribute your energy throughout your body using long strokes.
7. Then rest, breathe calmly, and tense your PC muscle.
8. Continue to closely observe the course of your arousal and stop at the right time. Continue to convey your emotions and the state of your arousal to your partner.

9. If you want, reward yourself at the end with a Big Draw, a distribution of energy, or an ejaculation, noting when, how, and where you feel it. Have fun!

If you allow yourself to feel at a deeper level—whatever it is that you feel—you will experience an orgasmic wave streaming through you in a very subtle way, spreading peace and happiness as you gently surf the waves of ecstasy.

MALE MENOPAUSE

While women are used to dealing with recurring cycles throughout their childbearing years, men primarily experience one single, large cycle: from youth to "andropause"—the male counterpart to the female menopause—which occurs with age.

Today's worship of youth leads to a fear of growing old and the changes associated with aging. While hormones bubble over in our youth and sexual energy calls for release, the sexual desires of older men begin to fade noticeably. The average male reaches the climax of his sexual potential at about 20 years of age. Statistics show a strong decrease in hormone levels (especially DHEA and testosterone) between the ages of 40 and 50. At age 55, about one in three men have testosterone levels of less than 3.5 ng/ml blood. This is a level so low that it is referred to as *hypogonadism*, a condition associated with difficulties in becoming sexually active.

A study in the US showed that 52 percent of men between the ages of 40 and 70 have dealt with problems related to their potency. While the average frequency of intercourse is about four to five times per month for men between the ages of 40 and 50, and three times per month among men 50 to 60, 25 percent of men in both these age brackets reported having no intercourse at all.

Men who do not consciously use their lingams begin to lose elasticity in the lingam tissue. This can result in erections that develop less quickly and less spontaneously. The penis may be less stiff even during erection, and the angle is usually flatter. It thus requires more, longer, and better physical stimulation to achieve an erection.

Estimates suggest that about 15 percent of men over 50 are chronically impotent. However, in most cases this loss of libido is not primarily caused by a lack of testosterone. Instead, it is often due to a mature man's inability to understand his evolving sexuality. When men are no longer as hormonally driven and excited as in previous years, it doesn't mean that their sexual time has passed. It simply means that their sexuality is transforming into a more mature form. To reject this experience would be as foolish as admiring the flowers on a tree in spring, but ignoring its wonderful fruit in the fall.

If a man thinks he has to show the same hormonal pressure in bed as a young man would, this would likely amplify any latent fears of failure and lead not only to erection problems, but to a complete rejection of sexuality. Viagra, the magic blue pill, is an attempt to compensate for this decrease in sexual vitality that comes with age. However, if we celebrated our maturity instead, we would gain a new understanding of the truly unique kind of potency that comes with maturity.

We continue to hear from men who deal with their midlife crises consciously, and who have found themselves able to enjoy sexuality and intimacy with their partners—as well as their orgasms—in a much deeper way. They report that they are much more able to let go than before. Mature men often have many fewer taboos than young men, and are more willing to try new things, which gives their sexual experiences a greater fullness.

Most women reach the climax of their sexual desire at around forty years of age—noticeably later than men. For some men and women this becomes a problem, rather than a chance to use what increasing maturity has to offer. If we clearly recognize the advantages, we may note that the differing receptiveness of men and women during their lives is not a joke that the gods are playing on us, but rather hides a secret of nature: what is initially an urge becomes a position of sexual attention during our later years. As we mature, our sexuality develops a more social component, a stronger feeling of belonging together, independent of sexual stimuli.

Age offers mature men the opportunity to develop the more feminine side of their sexuality, which may be driven by estrogen. Growing experience, tenderness, empathy, and stamina more than compensates for whatever may have been lost in spontaneity. Since mature men are not as fixated on a quick release, an extended lingam massage is an ideal way to precede a fulfilling love act. As we will see, the lingam massage opens an entirely new area in which we can enjoy our sexuality—an area that revolves around consciousness rather than youthful vitality.

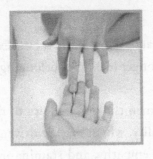

2
Energetic
and Spiritual Basics

THE TAOIST PHILOSOPHY OF
THE FIVE ELEMENTS

If we limit our sexuality to the physical experience, we see only the tip of the iceberg and will not appreciate its immense hidden depths. The following chapter offers practical exercises for deepening your understanding and helping you refine your sexual experiences. It offers a guide to discovering the infinite energetic potential that resides within each of us.

The energetic and spiritual qualities of lingam massage are best explained by the ancient philosophy of Taoism. At the center of Taoist teaching is the balance between the male and female principles; not worship of either polarity, but an appreciation of both. According to Taoist teaching, the entire world came into being when the original energy, Wu-Chi, split into a male principle (yang) and a female principle (yin). Yin and yang are two opposing, but not exclusionary, principles that could not exist without each other—without man, no woman; without day, no night, and so on.

According to Taoist teaching, yin and yang are present to different degrees in all people, animals, plants, events, and even in objects. Growth and harmony lie in finding balance between these two polarities, not in destroying one in favor of the other. In this way, the encounter between a man and a woman during intercourse is more a question of nourishing and interacting, than one of simply creating and releasing tension.

In current Western thought, orgasm is often viewed as a climax after which everything is over. But if we look at the cycles of nature and see how the opposites of night and day and winter and summer play with one another, we understand that polarities are linked to one another in a sort of dance. A look into our own lives confirms that change, growth, and aging happen in waves. The saying "the path is the destination," captures this—Taoism is concerned not with reaching the destination as quickly as possible, but with enjoying the journey. And at every destination the next part of the journey awaits us. If we remember to appreciate the cyclical nature of things and the interactions between the pairs of opposites during a lingam massage, then arousal (yang) and relaxation (yin), become complementary parts of a new awareness. Over time this new awareness extends to other areas of our lives as well.

While the philosophy of Taoism is based on the pair of yin and yang, it does not present these ideas in terms of contradictions or extremes. Because each polarity always contains a little of the other, contradictions in the circle of life are always relative and never absolute—every viewpoint has its alternatives embedded somewhere within it. This applies also to our desire, no matter how strong or weak, subtle or animalist it may be at any one point. To know this can support us in accepting ourselves as we are.

The polarities of yin and yang can help us to understand the lingam massage with more subtlety. While it is obvious that the lingam is yang compared to a man's anus, which is more yin, even these designations are relative. For example, a man's chest is yin in relation to his back, but yang in relation to his stomach.*

The lingam massage itself contains stages of yin and yang. They are not fixed, but subject to constant transformation. Thus a man may sometimes feel receptive, which is a yin quality (for example when his prostate is touched and caressed), and then again dynamic (for example when his erect lingam is massaged). If you permit this ongoing evolution without pushing toward a particular destination right away, you will understand that the lingam massage is carried on a wave that is larger than yourself.

The changing experience during a lingam massage can be compared to the different seasons. The middle of summer represents the highest yang, the middle of winter the deepest yin. On the way from one to the other we cross all four seasons: spring (with a rising yang), summer (full yang), fall (rising yin) and winter (full yin).

Taoist teachings assign elements to these four seasons: Wood for spring (when trees begin to grow), Fire for summer (the sun burns), Metal for fall (when nature lets go) and Water for winter (nature relaxes like water in a lake).

The curve also shows the orgasm as a valley. We begin in the Wood phase as we give ourselves the space to feel our bodies and gradually expand. Then our arousal builds (Fire), breathing deepens and we begin to let go (Metal), until we fall into deepest relaxation, the valley of orgasm (Water).

Using this model, we can see that a person who simply wants to reach a quick climax during lingam massage will only experience one part of the wave, without savoring the descent from the Fire. Such a quick orgasm is perfectly fine, but lingam massage teaches that there are pleasures to be found beyond the first crest of the wave.

What makes the valley orgasm special is that the Fire of sexual arousal does not immediately shoot out, but is instead transformed by our awareness and intention into a valley curve. Tantric writings from

---

*See Michaela Reidl's *Yoni Massage* for more information on yin and yang parts of the body.

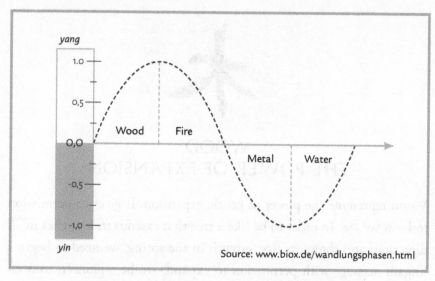

Fig. 2.1. The seasons as transformative phases

thousands of years ago say, "Begin by focusing attention on the growing fire. And by continuing it, avoid ashes at the end."[1]

The moment that is important is the one in which we transmute Fire into Metal, moving from yang to yin and from arousal into the valley orgasm. This point, when yang becomes yin, is accorded a fifth element—Earth. Earth itself is not a transformation phase, but a reference point that enables us to experience the other elements as transformation phases. The element Earth also represents the observer, the here and now, and the ability to dive into the valley orgasm even at the point of highest arousal. According to the Taoism of love it is the melding of the five elements—experiencing the connection of all of these states—that is decisive for our vitality, joy of life, health, happiness, and of course for a fulfilling sexuality.[2]

The philosophy of the five elements is based on the belief that all elements are equally important, and that each element wants to express itself within us. We experience harmony when these elements are in balance within us and appropriately expressed. That is why lingam massage is very different from masturbation—it is a dance with the elements that has neither beginning nor end.

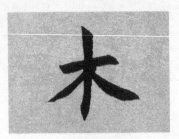

WOOD
THE POWER OF EXPANSION

Wood represents the power of gentle expansion. It gives us permission to be as we are. In order to be like a tree that extends its branches in all directions and shows its first growth in the spring, we need to begin a lingam massage with permission to expand—to be a pioneer, to overcome stagnation, and to enter unknown territory. For that reason it is important to create comfort and an open and pleasant atmosphere. When we are waiting for something pleasant, our attention relaxes and we open ourselves so as to better enjoy the coming pleasure. For this we have to be able to feel ourselves and grant ourselves permission to give in to this experience. Thus, the growth of the branches and of the tree becomes a metaphor for the sensory feelers within us.

It is helpful to begin a lingam massage—whether you are the giver or the receiver—by collecting yourself and gently stretching from your center. This creates an internal power that can later nourish the fire within. Just as trees gather their strength in the spring to nourish the growing buds that later explode into flowers and fruits, we begin the lingam massage with exercises to gather our strength.

▲ Humming as Stimulation

Humming creates a pulsation within the body that helps us touch our innermost selves. It carries a gentle wave of pleasure through all the tissues of the body, including the lingam, anus, and prostate. In this way, humming is a kind of vibrating massage from the inside that you can give yourself. Before the external massage, you can use humming to massage your insides. "Humming opens you. It opens your heart, your brain, and expands your ability to experience what is perceptible in a broader and deeper way."[3] Instead of being aware of your body, your body becomes aware of you.*

1. Assume a position in which you can comfortably sit for some time without moving. Begin humming into yourself in a fluid, unstructured manner and feel how the sound wave finds its natural path through your body. Feel whether there is resistance to this wave in any part of your body. Feel how your consciousness gently finds a path through your entire body and expands within it. Try to touch yourself from the inside—lovingly and without stress—in a tender self-stimulation.

2. You can also hum to your chakras, which are your body's energy centers. This puts your body into a state of gentle expansion that is an excellent preparation for lingam massage. To do this, lie down on your back, place your hands on your pubic bone, and direct your hum to the palms of your hands. After a few minutes, place your hands on your hara, the energy center that is located about two finger-widths beneath the navel. Hum under your hands here. Then place your hands on the solar plexus and hum there. Follow this by humming into your spiritual heart at the center of your chest, then into your throat, and finally into your forehead. For each of these, you can place your hands on that part of your body, or let them rest at your sides. If you want, you can support the chakra humming with a meditation CD.†

▲ Humming to Harmonize with Your Massage Partner

If you are about to have a lingam massage with a partner, humming together is one of the easiest ways to build an energetic bridge between

---

*For example, Osho's *Chakra Sounds Meditation*.
†You may want to have background music playing during this exercise. Try Tambura music, or the music of Dokuho and Juha Varpio.

you. The two partners may have very different temperaments, or be coming from very different work environments, so it is helpful to have ways of harmonizing their energies. This will make the subsequent massage much more enjoyable for both partners.

1. Sit down with your partner. The person who will receive the lingam massage begins humming. Let's say this is you. Now your partner tunes in to the humming wave in your body. He or she is sitting there in the most open and unprejudiced way that you can imagine. After a few minutes, your partner will feel that your humming is sending messages to his or her body; just as pendulum clocks in the same room tend to synchronize their rhythms, so to will humans—if they are open to doing so.

2. As soon as your partner is able to feel your humming wave in her body, she begins accompanying it with her hand along your body. She listens to the hum under her hand and notes whether there are obstacles to the wave at any point; if she finds any, she places her hand on them and begins humming into the spot with you in a targeted way to resolve any blockages.

3. Now hum into your lingam. It is not enough just to think about it, but important that you really *feel* your lingam from the inside as you hum. Feel how the sound wave reaches your lingam and make an effort to hum through any obstacles that it may encounter on its way. You can do this by yourself or with the help of your partner. If humming is not sufficient to penetrate these obstacles, try tapping them gently. Ideally, the sound wave will stream through your entire body, including your lingam.

4. Now imagine that it isn't you humming, but your lingam. Experience its fine vibrations and gentle expansion. Now hum into your testicles, and feel how this energizes them. Feel the river of strength that rises within you from your testicles. Now hum along your perineum until you reach your anus. Hum into your anus, making sure that it is really vibrating from the inside. If necessary, tap your anus gently

and feel how it lets go. Now feel inside your anus and feel the spot where the anus touches the prostate. Energize it with your humming and feel how the prostate vibrates with the sound wave. Then allow your hum to continue spreading throughout your body. Feel where it travels and accompany it without judging. If you want, you can now switch between humming and gentle sounds. Enjoy feeling your body from the inside.

▲ Body Flow Exercise

Humming represents the yin side of the Wood element. It brings you into touch with yourself and thus creates the preconditions for moving into the yang side of the element, expression through dance. The consciousness of your body that you experienced during humming now takes visible shape through the so-called "body flow." This term was coined at the Esalen institute and draws on the work of Mihaly Csikszentmihalyi, who researched the happiness-inducing effects of the state of harmony he called Flow.[4] "Body flow is contact with the intuitive consciousness of the body, expressed through motion."[5] In this, you learn to recognize and allow yourself to be moved by a wave of energy—an optimal preparation for enjoying a lingam massage.

1. Stand erect with plenty of space around you. Close your eyes, hold still, and feel inside yourself. Feel the ground under your feet, feel your breath, feel the sounds of your surroundings, feel how the sounds hit your skin. Feel your skin, the border of your body. Open yourself to your surroundings. Imagine that all the space around you is inside you and that you are filled with space.

2. When you are ready, turn on music that you like* and feel how the music penetrates through you. Imagine that the music is inside you and allow yourself to be moved by the music. Just as you neither forced nor suppressed your humming, you don't need to force or

---

*Suggestion for background music: Georg Deuter, *Nataraj*.

suppress any movements. Move gently while standing. Allow your movements to flow entirely from their own will. Feel the energies within you and give expression to them. Feel how your body responds to the energies of your surroundings. Your movements may begin gently at first and may grow more expressive bit by bit. If you like, you can keep your eyes closed.

There is no "I" in body flow that decides from the head how you move and what you want to look like for others. Your body moves by itself, and you are "only" its witness. You are in touch with your body's intelligence and being. Allow it to express itself, allow this permeability, allow the energies of the music and your surroundings to move around inside you. Experience how you become a single wave of energy that expresses itself through dance like a single wave amidst an ocean. If you want, you can play with sometimes taking control of the movements before letting them go again.

You can also experience body flow without music and simply let yourself be moved by the energies of your surroundings.

▪ Body Flow with a Partner

Body flow with a partner is a particularly nice way to prepare for a lingam massage. Together you create the space for the coming experience.

1. Stand facing each other and hold hands. Feel the ground under your feet, the borders of your skin.
2. Now picture the boundaries between you dissolving as you become nothing but space.
3. Now begin with the body flow, moving in harmony with your partner. Experience how doing this melts two forms of energy into one being.
4. When you feel that you are dancing as one being, let go of one hand, then the other, and allow whatever movements come to you.

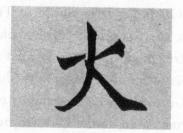

FIRE
THE POWER OF SAYING "YES"

According to Chinese medicine, the Fire element corresponds to the heart. This means that the key to our Fire energy rests in our physical and spiritual heart—the material for it is our embrace of life. In this way, we can picture our hearts saying "yes" to life with every beat. This "yes" includes respect for our own desires and needs, the readiness to stand up for ourselves, and a willingness to say yes to everything in and about ourselves, even when others might not agree.

Fire also has a yin and a yang side. On the inside we feel our heart and are connected to its beat and to the larger life that comes through us. This is Fire's yin aspect. Its yang aspect is arousal.

The willingness to enter and explore uncharted territory, which we developed with the Wood element, strengthens our Fire and makes it possible for us to burn *for* something. It takes great skill to keep the fire burning, and this is an endeavor that can include both fantasies and role-play. That is why Joseph Kramer, the founder of lingam massage, emphasizes time and again how important it is to enter the role of the "sexual masseur."

Saying Yes

Sometimes we find it difficult to say yes to our sexuality or to intimate massage. The enlightened yogini Yeshe Tsogyel* can be a great inspiration in this regard. She was the companion of the Guru Rinpoche

---

*Yeshe = "wisdom from the beginning of time," Tsogyel = "queen of the ocean-gliding quality of the soul."

(Padmasambhava), who brought Buddhism to Tibet. In the monastery where she lived, she was often sexually molested by the monks living there. After struggling with these repeated assaults, she eventually decided to see her own mirror image in the lusting monks and to accept them, since Guru Rinpoche had emphasized to her that "yes" was the most important word on the spiritual path. She let go of her thoughts of how immoral and improper the advances were, and ceased judging the people who made them. This changed the situation entirely. In a moment of satori (an event of enlightenment), she was shaken by a laughter that tore apart all dualistic concepts. After that, she radiated a presence that made it impossible for the monks to approach her without her consent. From Yeshe Tsogyel we learn not only unconditional acceptance, but also optimism and the power to transform things through our "yes."

Fire is also related to the readiness to sacrifice oneself, just as flame consumes itself. We sacrifice our comfort, our constructs and dualistic concepts, in order to allow ourselves to burn. To be in the fire of enthusiasm means saying "yes" to whatever it is that life brings you, to celebrate everything.

Of course, this doesn't mean that you are not entitled to reject something and say "no." If your "no" is true, you should stand by it. But before you say it, make sure that your "no" is authentic, and not a reaction based on moralistic concepts, fear, or inhibition. Do not allow an inauthentic "no" to prevent you from becoming aroused. Perhaps the following lines can inspire you.

The Healthiest Word in the World

YES. You should cut out YES and hang it on your wall. So that YES can imprint itself in your mind. YES functions like this: think YES if at some time you are not in the mood. Because *no* keeps you always subject to your moods. Think YES if sometimes you don't have an erection. *No* only makes you frustrated and doesn't solve any problems (unless you want to feel sorry for yourself). Think YES if your body is tense. Saying "Oh, I'm so tense," won't help. Say YES to problems with feelings. To problems with intimacy. To problems in bed. Because *no* won't save the day. Say YES to your experience with lingam massage, because who knows all the good things that can come of it? Say YES to a prostate or anal massage, even if you have never had one before.

YES is medicine. Better than liquids or powders. YES helps in the long run. YES stimulates your circulation. It makes your heart happy. It shrinks your worries. It warms your life. YES should be your philosophy, but it is hard to learn. Once you have learned, pass it on, YES?

Because we sometimes carry our hearts in our mouths, the Fire element is also linked to speech. If you talk with your partner about the things you say "yes" to, and the things you say "no" to, you will activate the Fire within. "Once we feel our needs and desires and express them, we unleash the Fire within ourselves and our partners."[6]

▲ *Heart Encounter*

1. Sit down facing your partner. Take a few deep breaths together, then feel into your hearts—your own and your partner's. Allow yourselves to be in your hearts. Allow feelings, sensations, emotions, and especially desires and needs to be noted. Ask yourself: "How do I feel, what do I wish for, what do I desire, what do I need right now?" Share the answers with your partner as directly and clearly as possible. When speaking, make sure to remain in touch with

your heart and avoid drifting off into projections and imaginations. Maintain respect for yourself and for your partner. As a listener, make sure to open yourself as widely as possible to what your partner is trying to tell you.*

2. This exercise is not about your partner fulfilling your needs, but more about being able to share what is in your heart and have your partner listen with an open heart. This strengthens the joint Fire of your hearts. During the course of the conversation, this Fire burns toxins and overcomes stereotypes and old feelings. As you speak, your sexual desires may change. You may begin to discover things that were completely unknown at the beginning of your conversation. For example, if you speak with your partner before the lingam massage, you may feel a wish to try a prostate or anal massage. Or it may be that the desire to ejaculate will give way to curiosity about the Big Draw.

3. Without these exchanges, your love life may become rigid. You have to share your feelings and needs, and if you can do this in an honest, authentic, and true way—without hiding or holding back—you will discover how this creates intimacy between you and your partner. Such intimacy will improve your love life and your experience with lingam massage later on.

Celebrating, Shaking, Dancing

While the yin side of Fire is about saying yes—speaking, and sharing—the yang side is about celebrating, shaking, and dancing. What is lingam massage if not a celebration of your lingam and a big dance? You don't need a reason or an occasion to celebrate your life and yourself. Celebration is a state of mind, independent of circumstances, and one that is important for the Fire of the heart. You can simply celebrate your masculinity. Let us use the power of "yes" to bring Fire to your pelvic region.

*More exercises like this one can be found in Carol Hwoschinsky's *Listening with the Heart* (Indianola, Wash.: Compassionate Listening Project, 2002).

▲ Yes-Yes Exercise

1. Stand up, with legs slightly apart. Hold your hands in front of your lower body, as if they were holding a horizontal pipe.
2. Now move your pelvis rhythmically forward, while at the same time moving your hands down toward your pelvis, and loudly call out "Yes!"
3. Then swing your pelvis and arms back again.

Repeat the exercise about twenty times. Then take a break, feel inside yourself, and enjoy the fire that is spreading through your pelvis.

▲ Hey-Yes Exercise

1. Stand up as before, with your legs slightly apart.
2. Squat down, moving your buttocks and arms toward the ground and call out "Hey!"
3. Stand erect, lift your arms above your head (making your body form a Y), and call out "Yes!"

Repeat this exercise about twenty times. This exercise energizes your whole body, and is especially powerful if done with a partner. (For this, stand facing your partner.)

To continue stoking the fire, take every opportunity to dance. If Wood was about the movement of gentle expansion (body flow), Fire is an invitation to move wildly and passionately.* This exercise can be experienced even more deeply if you first shake off everything that is constricting you.

▲ Shaking Meditation

Drums make good background music for this exercise, for example Osho's Kundalini Meditation, *Laughing Drums*.

---

*A guided dance meditation can be found on the CD *Coming Alive, A Dance Meditation* by Krish and Amana (Learning Love Institute).

1. Stand with your feet shoulder-width apart and your knees slightly bent. Steady yourself with one hand against a wall or your partner.
2. Now place your weight on one leg while shaking the other. Feel the relaxation rising up through your calf. Relax your knee, your thigh, and your hip.
3. Place this leg back on the floor and compare it with the other. Feel into both legs. Which one is longer, lighter, better circulated?
4. Now shake the other leg.
5. Return to the standing position, and begin moving your knees, causing your body to shake forward and back. Move your pelvis and arms together with your knees, and allow your elbows and wrists to shake, as well as your head, shoulders, and back. Let your mouth fall open and your breathing deepen. If sounds come out, like moans or sighs, that's okay.
6. Allow the shaking to envelop your entire body, even the inside. Heart, stomach, liver, and kidneys can all shake. Feel whether you have tension anywhere in your body—especially in your perineum or lingam—and allow it to resolve.
7. Feel the energy rise upward from your feet and continue to let the "I" go as you shake. Experience your body shaking by itself, as you witness it. Don't compel the shaking or suppress it.

Picture your body as made of sand, with everything becoming fine and flowing as it shakes. Enjoy the shaking that your body is offering you. The flow will resolve spiritual and physical tensions. Shaking encompasses and energizes every cell of your body; every cell vibrates along with its neighbor.

As shaking stimulates your metabolism, blood begins to flow; toxins are released and your body's diaphragms relax and renew themselves. Whenever you feel tired, stiff, or tense, you can use this shaking exercise to relax and energize yourself. But there is another special reason that shaking is so important:

Occasionally, you can experience a full-body orgasm during lingam massage; when this happens your whole body is grasped by a deep, liberating shaking. This is an expression of the rising life energy that is making its way through your chakras during a full-body orgasm. Once you have learned to allow yourself to be shaken by your body, you can double your enjoyment of this kind of orgasm. Additionally, you and your partner can both shake yourselves while you make love—just give it a try.

A discreet alternative to shaking is bouncing. You can do this at your desk, at the bus stop, or ideally on a medicine ball or trampoline. Bouncing every once in a while helps you reduce tension and improve your circulation. It's also lots of fun.

▲ Dance

And then dance. Dance may be the first and oldest human form of expression. Among traditional Native American people, for example, dance remains as important as eating, drinking, or sleeping, and is still an essential part of everyday life.

The type of dancing that we recommend here is not about looking good, but about expressing your feelings and impulses through movement. If you are feeling angry, dance anger, and if you feel like celebrating, then celebrate yourself in dance.

To begin, you can build on the body flow of the Wood element. Close your eyes and feel the music touching your body. Don't move yet, just feel the music with your whole body. When you're ready, begin to dance, to celebrate, and perhaps at one point even to explode. Or you can simply put on exhilarating music and dance wildly, without stopping first—as you prefer.

Perhaps you want to experiment by alternating between closed eyes and open ones, or dancing with half-closed eyes. If the fire of enthusiasm takes hold within you, you can express it through sound, calling out "hey," "ya," "yippie," or whatever you feel like. Whether you are bouncing or dancing, make sure to let your body do the "work." Without suppressing or forcing anything, allow yourself to be "danced."

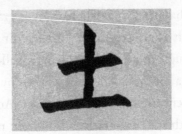

EARTH
THE STRENGTH OF OPENNESS

The Earth stands at the center of all life and thus symbolizes centeredness, originality, and the strength to be in the here and now. Earth allows us to trust in life and to remain open and relaxed. These qualities enable us to realize our true potential.

If we get lost in drama, melancholy, self-pity, or dreams instead of recognizing reality, we lose our presence and the perception of our true identity. On the other hand, if we are hard and judgmental of others, those around us will lose their openness. This can happen if we judge someone before giving him a massage, for instance, instead of accepting him as he is: maybe he doesn't look the way we want him to, or maybe he doesn't have an erection. Similarly, the recipient of a lingam massage should forego making judgments about himself or his partner, since these will block large components of the experience.

Of course, you can and should tell your partner if something happens during a massage that is uncomfortable for you, but don't give in to judgments that don't concern your immediate well-being. This massage is about perceiving what is happening to you free of pictures from the past and projections about others.

▲ Loving Eye Contact

1. Sit across from your partner and look each other in the eyes, with your mouths slightly open. If you experience tensions, judgments, or distracting thoughts, recognize them and label them in your head as "tension," "judgment," or "thought"—but do not pursue them further.

2. Now close your eyes, lean forward slightly until your heads touch at the forehead. If you want, you can have your hands touch too. Perceive your partner without judgment and with an open heart.

3. After a while, break the physical connection of forehead and hands, but continue feeling your connection to each other. Practice seeing your partner without judgments or influences from the past. Allow your glance to become softer until the contours blur. This may or may not change the way you see the face of your partner, but the important thing is the innocent, unbiased look that honors your partner as he or she is. As you get more practice, you will feel more closeness and connection.

Looks can kill, hurt, or freeze people—think of the look of Medusa. But looks can also convey trust, openness, and relaxation. And these are exactly the qualities that are part of the Earth element. Only trust and openness can allow what is larger than you and your partner to work through you.

Openness, Trust, Enabling

Openness means allowing people and things to be as they are, foregoing control over them. We cannot try to control our partner and then expect to have uncontrolled, beautiful orgasms during lovemaking or lingam massage. Control and openness do not go together. Openness means accepting a partner and all that he or she entails. This creates the basis for our partners to show their more expansive sides.

Another aspect of the Earth element is trust. Trust means not forcing or suppressing anything. Let's take an example from nature: once we have sown seeds and are waiting for our plants to bloom, there is no point in pulling on the buds and stems. Applied to lingam massage, this means that if a partner does not have an erection or pleasant feelings, it doesn't help—in fact, it's counterproductive—to tell him to enjoy himself, or to try harder. It is just as futile if you try harder yourself by rubbing him up and down. Instead, create openness, and trust that everything will come out all right in the end. By doing so, we allow all insecurities to leave us during lingam massage. We will feel ready to experience whatever arises.

Earth element also represents persistence; we persist in wanting to be as we are. This gives us the possibility of letting other people be as they are. Then we can feel like ourselves in the here and now. When we are fully present, we can experience an "I am" moment that will always be true. Allowing this true being, the true "I am," is the yang component of Earth. It is said that Socrates would regularly go to the market and talk to the uneducated slaves that were being sold there. In these conversations, he prompted them to say words of highest wisdom. He was able to do this by speaking to their highest potential, by empowering them.

Just as Socrates enabled slaves to achieve high wisdom, you can empower your partner to reach great lovemaking, just by being relaxed, open, and present. According to tantric teachings, gods can appear through lovers. Lingam massage offers one way of helping men feel god. At the same time, you can feel god or goddess working through you, guiding your hands, and moving your partner into ecstasy. The secret of empowering lies in recognizing the highest potential in the other, and awakening it.

▲ Empowering the Senses

If you like, you can record this guided meditation and listen to it with your partner before a lingam massage.

1. Relax, and let go of all plans and goals. Open yourself to the present and to your own receptiveness. Move into a state of no resistance. If you experience tension or discomfort, accept it without judgment and allow it to leave your body as you exhale. Allow your thoughts to become softer. Now turn your consciousness to the quiet that exists behind your thoughts and images, the infinite breadth of your true being.

2. Offer your hearing to the highest, most godly aspect within you. Perceive where your hearing comes from, and allow the highest elements within you to hear through you. Let your hearing continue to turn inward, listen to the subtle tones of your insides. Listen inside yourself and make yourself aware that the godly aspect inside you is now listening through you. Dedicate your hearing to the god or goddess within you.

3. Now turn your attention to your sense of vision. What do you see when you close your eyes? What shades, light reflections, visions? Perceive where your vision comes from, and allow the godly to see through you. Follow your vision to your origin. Dedicate your internal vision to the highest elements within yourself.

4. Now become aware of your sense of smell. What scents can you smell? Perceive where your smell comes from and allow the godly to smell through you. Follow your sense of smell to its origin. Dedicate your sense of smell to the highest elements within yourself.

5. Now become aware of your sense of taste. What do you taste? Perceive from what place your taste comes and allow the highest elements within yourself to taste through you.

6. Now become aware of your sense of touch. Feel your skin and the tissues of your body, become touch. Feel where your sense of touch is coming from and allow the highest elements within you to feel through you. Move your sense of touch deep to the inside, free from effort or resistance.

You now hear, see, smell, taste, and feel the godly through your senses. Again make yourself conscious of the inner place from which all of this is coming. Where does it come from? The origin of all these senses lies deep within you.

Receivers: Focus your attention on your lingam. Imagine the highest elements within you to be focusing on your lingam. Feel how these elements experience your lingam. Dedicate the senses of your lingam to the highest elements within yourself.

Givers: Focus your attention on your hands. Imagine that the highest elements within you are inside your hands, moving them to touch your partner. How does visualizing this feel for you?

Whether you are giving or receiving, you can experience the wholeness that comes from identification with the highest elements within you. Now gently return from your meditation.

Accepting the Lingam as It Is

Many men have separated their lingams from their sense of themselves. They speak of it like a third person, as if it were not truly part of them, saying, "He's not in the mood today . . ." The psychologist Stephen Wolinsky called this the "I'm not my body trance."[7] This separation may have its root in religious views of the flesh as sinful and therefore as something we should not identify ourselves with. But in fact our bodies are vehicles through which we can experience "higher" sensations, and we should therefore get to know them rather than reject them.

A separation of consciousness from the lingam also significantly reduces the pleasure from lingam massage: a man divided in this way is either in his head and unable to feel enough sexual fire to get an erection, or he focuses fully on his penis, forgetting the rest of his body in doing so, and ejaculating too quickly.

To enjoy a lingam massage, it is good to feel at one with your body, to accept it and its arousal (or lack thereof). If you can do this, your body will begin to communicate with you, and you will be able to live in harmony with it as a whole.

▲ Feeling the Lingam and Connecting Head, Heart, and Pelvis

1. With your eyes closed, and without touching your lingam, ask yourself: "Is there any way for me to know whether my lingam is there or not?" This question alone will focus your attention on your lingam and you will begin to feel inside it. How is it feeling? Is it filled with blood or empty? Is it tired or lively?

2. Once you can feel your lingam, you can feel any other body part too, and create a connection between them. So now focus your attention on your head area and ask your head: "What do you need to find peace?" Wait for the answer. Now feel into your heart and ask your heart: "What do you need to experience love?" Finally feel into your instincts, your animal nature that is located somewhere in your lower body, and ask it: "What do you need to experience vitality and strength?" In each case, wait for the answer.

Now you can connect the energy of Fire with that of Earth: connect the "Yes" of life with openness and awareness of the inside of your body.

▲ "Yes" Visualization for Lingam Massage

1. Picture yourself about to receive a lingam massage. Allow yourself to be as you are, and relax. Now allow the word *yes* to rise up from deep inside you, with both sound and feeling. Say "yes" to the coming lingam massage, "yes" to whatever you are about to experience. Speak, whisper, or think "yes, yes, yes." Then allow the sound of "yes" to enter your body. Feel how it reaches all the cells in your body, especially in your lingam. Yes, yes, yes . . .
2. After some time, make contact with your instincts, with your animalistic side. Say to it: "I want to be more in touch with you. You have been there for me all of my life and I have never fully accepted you. Is there something I can do for you so that we can work better together?" Then enter the silence and listen to what this part has to say. Then say, "Thank you," loudly.
3. Feel how the sound of "yes" is filling your lingam. "Yes, yes, yes." Begin talking to yourself: "Yes, yes, yes. I say 'yes' to myself, to my instincts, to my lingam. Yes, yes!" Breathe in freshness and truth. Perhaps your body wants to move, stretch—yes, yes! And when you are ready to open your eyes, feel completely awake and conscious.

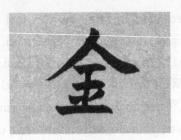

METAL
THE STRENGTH OF COURAGE

Metal is the ore that must be discovered and extracted from the ground through active effort. If you want to dig for your own inner metal, your hidden (sexual) potential, you have to descend deep into your subconscious. Searching for your inner metal will require both courage and stamina. To get metal flowing we have to heat it up, since it only becomes usable through strong fire.

While Wood symbolizes stimulation, Fire arousal, and Earth harmonization, Metal is about transformation. This transformation happens in two steps: first, we have to dig for the core, our hidden sexual selves, below the surface of our sexual identity. We have to be able to name and accept what we find there. The second step is about refining our inner true nature by placing it into the furnace of Fire, and giving it our trust so that it can reveal its true face.

In this process Metal also includes the strength to differentiate. Like a sharp sword, it stands for clarity, recognition, and consciousness. We recognize what is part of us and what is not, and we are able to leave behind anything we no longer need. In its untransformed state, Metal can lead us toward control, prejudice, or condemnation. To protect us from possible attacks from the outside, the Metal element wants to prevent anything negative, shameful, or unpleasant from surfacing. This can extend to a general resistance to any kind of change. Unconscious fears may make us rigid, hard, compulsive, and controlling.

In our journey to our hidden sexual selves we will rarely encounter pure gold. Instead, we will usually find a mixture of light and shadow, of gold and toxins. We have to accept both in order to have deeper sexual experiences. This means that we have to put all aspects of our sexuality into the furnace of our consciousness—even those we might normally be ashamed of. Such consciousness symbolizes the courage of the Metal element.

The Hidden Sexual Self

Many people wear masks without being aware of it. They act in ways they believe they are supposed to act, and feel what they believe they are supposed to feel. This also applies to sexual acts and feelings; many men have "sexualized" their responses to their lingams, because they believe that is what they are supposed to do. Since lingam massage is not primarily designed to stimulate arousal, however, but to get in touch with direct sexual feelings, we sometimes have to dig beyond the sexualized notions about the lingam to discover the gold deposits within ourselves.

Your true sexual self lives under your masks and dogmas. It reveals itself only when it feels accepted and able to breathe. Each of us has such a sexual self, even if we are unaware of it. If we do not experience ourselves as sexual beings it is often because we are hiding our true sexual nature from ourselves and others.

Our hidden sexual selves include parts of us that we have locked up in our subconscious—parts we do not want to look at, and about which we know relatively little. These are the parts we are ashamed of, that we do not want to show to others. But it is only with these hidden parts that we can recognize our true needs and desires and thereby free ourselves from fears, expectations, and imagination. That doesn't mean that we have to fully realize all the wishes of this part of ourselves—it rather means that we have to accept them, and put them into the furnace of our consciousness along with our (sexual) masks.

▲ Access to Your Hidden Sexual Self

Begin by answering the following questions, as honestly as possible.

1. **Childhood:** Think back to the first time that you felt something like sexual arousal. How old were you when you had sexual fantasies

for the first time? What do you recall of them? What were the circumstances? Was the situation pleasant or unpleasant?

2. **Sexual highs and lows:** Revisit some of your past sexual encounters. Then concentrate on one that was particularly arousing for you, and another that you found particularly difficult. Describe these encounters in as much detail as you like. Why were these encounters so important for you?

3. **Erotic fantasies:** Imagine that you want to become sexually aroused and can use any fantasy you would like to this end. Think about everything that you know about your fantasies and describe the one that will arouse you most quickly. Describe the climax, the point of highest arousal in the fantasy. What makes the fantasy so arousing?

4. **Goal orientation:** Ask yourself: what do I want to experience in my sexuality or in a lingam massage? What potential improvement do I hope for in comparison to my current state?

Once again, make yourself aware of all the images and scenes that relate to your hidden sexual self, especially those that are difficult for you. Now place them in the furnace of your consciousness to release the sexual potential, the pure life energy that is trapped within them. Do this by saying the following reconciliation formula: "Even if I _____, I accept myself fully and completely!" Complete the blank in the sentence by filling in the fantasy you are working with.

Continue repeating this formula while following an imaginary figure eight with your eyes, until you feel that your internal energy system has created a deep relaxation and relief. Alternatively, you can move your eyes rapidly from left to right and back again instead of drawing the figure eights. Since the orientation of our pupils is closely connected with the functioning of our brains, the movement of the eyes ensures that our reconciliation formula reaches all regions of the brain.

The "trick" of the reconciliation formula is in its built-in transformation mechanism: if a fantasy, imagination, or mask is unpleasant, destructive, or burdensome, it is resolved through the formula. But if it is positive for you, it becomes even stronger. It is your subconscious that differentiates between the two. Of course you can use this reconciliation formula at other times as well, for example when you are afraid to give in to a lingam massage, if you are encountering a blockage, or feel restricted from practicing the Big Draw. In those cases, simply say: "Although I have this hesitation about _____, I accept myself fully and completely.

Conscious Breathing
An important instrument and great supporter of our consciousness is our breath. It is for this reason that traditions of yoga and tantra have been exploring breathing practices for millennia.

- ▲ **Conscious deep breathing has a vitalizing function:** A single deep breath provides about seven times as much oxygen as a shallow one.
- ▲ **Breathing is energizing:** Even fifteen minutes of conscious breathing can have a positive effect on your metabolism.
- ▲ **Breathing is detoxifying:** Deep breathing will increase lymph activity tenfold.
- ▲ **Breathing is life:** Humans can only survive for a few minutes without breathing.
- ▲ **Breathing is cleansing:** 70 percent of all waste materials are excreted through breathing, 20 percent via the skin, and only 10 percent through the digestive system.
- ▲ **Breathing can be increased:** The average person usually uses only about 20 percent of their lung capacity.

At this point we want to focus on two kinds of breathing that are important during lingam massage: conscious breathing and energizing breathing.

Conscious breathing means that you are conscious of your own breath. Turning your attention to your breath is the easiest way to connect with your inner self at most times in life. Conscious breathing helps you to not drift away during lingam massage. As the recipient of a massage you will encounter a wide range of different stimuli. At the same time, the temptation is great to let your attention drift away from your body, away from the here and now, and into various fantasies. By returning your attention to your breathing, you remain conscious.

This also applies if you are giving a lingam massage. If both partners are breathing consciously, you will create a breathing bridge that keeps you both in living contact. As Joseph Kramer said to one client: "If you stop breathing, I will stop touching you!" If your consciousness remains in your breath, you will be able to remain relaxed even in highly erotic situations, and will thus be able to enjoy them consciously.

▲ Feeling Your Breath

1. Assume a comfortable position and relax. Exhale deeply and allow the inhalation to proceed by itself. Then simply continue to observe your breathing. Don't force it or suppress it. Feel how your breathing happens, here and now. Trust your breath.

2. Now begin to feel your entire body as it rests here. Feel yourself from head to toe, left to right, inside and out. Become aware of your body as the unity of an infinite number of functions that you can trust in. It is a miracle within which you are at home. Because energy follows attention, you can use your attention to steer your awareness wherever you wish, and can fill this region with energy.

▲ Feeling Electricity Under Your Skin

1. Again assume a position that is comfortable for you. Observe your breathing without suppressing or forcing it. While observing your breath, focus your attention on the sensations under your skin. Feel all the movements beneath your skin, perhaps like bubbles of sparkling water or wine, or like small needle pricks. Notice how this energy feels slightly different under the skin of your left and right hands. Different in each hand, in each finger, perhaps a little like

fine electricity. Continue breathing normally while observing all of this.

2. Now feel your heartbeat and the pulse of your blood in each finger. Feel the pulse under your skin, and how it feels slightly different in each hand and each finger. Compare your two hands, then your two pinkies, ring fingers, middle fingers, index fingers, and thumbs, and notice how each of them feels slightly different on the inside.

3. While continuing to observe these sensations, focus your concentration on your breath. Feel your inhalations and exhalations like small waves, like high tides that reach out to your fingertips before receding. Each breath is a wave of energy in your body. Also feel the gaps—the turning points between inhalation and exhalation, and between each exhalation and the next inhalation.

4. Now play with your attention. Concentrate for a while on the sensations under your skin, then on your pulse, and then on the breathing waves in your hands. With the next breath feel how the breathing wave flows through your entire body, from head to toes. Feel the flood tide when you inhale and the ebb tide when you exhale. Feel the pulsation in your ankles and in each of your toes. Feel the electricity prickling under your feet.

5. While your breath continues to flow in and out, concentrate your attention on your lingam and experience how the breathing wave flows all the way to its tip during inhalation, and leaves during exhalation. Also feel the turning point at the tip of your lingam and take good note of it. After a while, you can focus your attention on the breath that you clearly feel in the tip of your lingam. Concentrate on the feeling of your pulse and the prickling of electricity under your skin. Observe details that you may not have noticed before.

Each region you breathe into consciously is freed from constriction and rejuvenated. This allows you to easily reach the state of expanded consciousness that Joseph Kramer termed "sexual trance."

▲ Breathing during Lingam Massage

Playing with different breathing rhythms is an excellent preparation for lingam massage. Rhythmic breathing can also help you stay in the here and now during the massage, distributing your sexual energy through-out your body.

■ Rhythmic Full Breathing

Inhale deeply and with full effort, then relax while exhaling. The emphasis here is on the inhalation, since the exhalation will happen by itself. If you want, purse your lips as you inhale and make a noise as if you were sucking on a thick straw. Make sure that you inhale deeply, but remain relaxed. Enjoy a strong and rhythmic inhalation as if you were very happily sucking on something. Make sure not to pause too long between breaths, and to fully let go with each exhalation. This strong breathing awakens the senses, and floods the body with oxygen and energy. If you want, try moving your pelvis in harmony with the flow of your breath.*

Breathing in this way will help you circulate the erotic energy that builds up first in the genitals and then in the whole body during the course of a lingam massage. To do this, you simply have to focus your attention.

■ Variation A—Activating the Microcosmic Orbit

While inhaling, visualize your energy running from your genitals up along your back to your head and over your scalp. Then, as you exhale, visualize your energy running down along the front of your body back to your genitals.

■ Variation B—The Inner Flute

This is an alternative to the Microcosmic Orbit. As you inhale, imagine that your breathing reaches deep into all corners and gaps in your pelvis,

---

*The CD *Zen Gong* by Michael Vetter is good for background music, especially the first piece: "Pulsation Time."

your lingam, and your testicles. When you exhale, the energy that your breath brings in doesn't leave, but rather stays in the pelvis and each time rises a few inches upward along your spine. Continue breathing in this way for about five minutes, moving your energy upward bit by bit toward your head, until you imagine or perhaps even feel that your energy has reached your head and is now flowing into your pituitary gland.

▪ Variation C—The Straw

During inhalation, visualize yourself sucking sexual energy into your body through your lingam as though it were a snout or a straw, and draw all of this energy upward. Let it ebb a bit back toward the lingam during exhalation. With your next breath, again visualize sexual energy being drawn into your body through your lingam. This time it should stay a bit higher than before during the exhalation. Support this energizing breath by tensing your PC muscle as you inhale, and relaxing it as you exhale. (See page 37.) You can see that variant C is the opposite of variant B; our experience suggests that it is worth trying both and seeing which you prefer.

It is not important whether you choose the regular rhythmic full breathing or one of the variations. What matters are strong inhalations and letting everything go during exhalation. Simply try to see which feels best for you. Your breath will show you the way.

After you have been breathing deeply and rhythmically for about half an hour, you will note a feeling throughout your whole body that closely resembles a sexual orgasm. When you combine this feeling with lingam massage you can experience very pleasant sensations in your whole body. But it is best to begin practicing the breathing techniques separately, to gain comfort and a sense of familiarity with them.

▲ Synchronizing Breathing and Touch

When you are giving a lingam massage to someone else, you can guide and accompany your partner's breathing with your own.

Ask your partner to begin rhythmic full breathing with you. In your thoughts, connect your breath with the breath of your partner. Touch him and stroke your hands across his body. Combine your touch and, later, your lingam massage strokes, with joint rhythmic breathing. Touch your partner with the same consciousness you would use if you were touching yourself.

▲ Penis Breathing

When you are receiving a lingam massage—from yourself or someone else—it is helpful to work with your breathing before the massage begins.

1. Picture your lingam as a tube through which your breath flows. As you inhale, energy streams from the root of your lingam to its tip; as you exhale, it runs from the tip back to the root. Breathe like this for a few minutes without interruption. Continue to feel into your lingam more and more, as you have learned in the exercises for the Earth element (see page 86). Feel whether there are any parts of your lingam that are tense. This can happen especially in the center of the lingam root. If you discover tension here, relax from the inside while continuing to inhale and exhale rhythmically. Use your attention to explore every part of your lingam from the inside and relax it using your breathing.

2. Now give your breath a quality. You can, for example, picture your inhalation filling your lingam with liquid lava. Or you can breathe into your lingam a characteristic that is important to you in the moment. In the beginning, it is easiest to breathe "relaxation" into your lingam. Once you are able to do this, and are able to also feel "liquid lava" in your lingam, try "joyful arousal." Breathe "joyful arousal" into your lingam and observe whether and how this causes it to change. At the end, breathe "readiness for contact."

▲ Anal Breathing

Anal breathing is especially helpful if you are receiving an anal massage.

1. Assume a comfortable position and begin with rhythmic full breathing.
2. Now picture yourself breathing through your anus. Tense your anus while inhaling, and imagine drawing energy in through it. Direct this energy upward along your spine. Relax your anus muscle as you exhale and picture the energy flowing back a bit.
3. With the next inhalation, visualize the energy reaching slightly higher along your spine. Continue breathing in this way until the energy has reached your head.

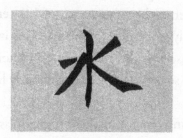

WATER
THE STRENGTH OF CALMNESS

Water is devotion. The rhythmic full breathing of the Metal element nourishes the devotion that is accessible through Water. Once you have breathed deeply and for long enough, a different experience suddenly becomes possible. We can call this larger experience god, Tao, strength of nature, holiness, or anything we want.

The nature of the Water element is relaxation. Water is entirely effortless; it does not try, but still always reaches its destination. Just think of streams and rivers that find their way to the sea entirely without effort. In the same way, deep relaxation is a precondition for making possible this larger thing, which we may also call orgasm, "petit mort," or mystical experience. Perhaps the easiest way to reach this state of relaxation is with a progressive muscle relaxation exercise. Indeed, the Big Draw that can end a lingam massage is in essence a synthesis of breathing ecstasy and progressive muscle relaxation.

More Pleasure and Depth through Progressive Muscle Relaxation

The lingam massage is structured in such a way as to promote relaxation and security for the receiver right from the beginning. This pleasant relaxation makes it possible to experience the sensual and erotic aspects of the massage. It builds up a strong energy that can then spread throughout your body. However, if you are too tense, the channels through which this energy can flow may be blocked. This will make it more difficult for you to experience an orgasm or to avoid premature ejaculation.

Instructions like "let go," or "give me your leg," will usually prompt the receiving partner to become aware of his tension and relax his muscles. But this only works for a moment. This is in part because the relaxation of the muscles is directed by the autonomic nervous system. In addition, modern society causes a continuously high level of stimulation and stress.

One frequent consequence of these high stress levels is waking up in the night and not being able to fall fully asleep again. The body continues to look for the state it is used to during daytime. Our daily experience no longer feeds into the main storage—our subconscious—which means that our daily consciousness can no longer be turned off. It remains stuck on a mid-level and keeps within it the events of the outside world. Our body cannot let go, and we experience muscle tensions, high blood pressure, and possible impotence. In this overheated state the fine sensitivity of our body gets lost, causing our sexuality and receptiveness to touch to suffer. Progressive muscle relaxation uses a trick that gradually enables us to experience truly deep relaxation: the conscious tensing and relaxing of individual muscle groups, followed by conscious attention to these parts. This stimulates stronger blood circulation, which the body registers as pleasant relaxation.

▲ Progressive Muscle Relaxation

1. Focus your attention on your right hand and note how it feels.
2. Consciously tense the muscles in your right hand by making a fist.

Tense the fist strongly enough to feel the tension, but not to feel pain.

3. Maintain the tension and observe it consciously, slowly counting to seven while continuing to breathe normally. Observe without judgment what is happening in the tensed muscles.

4. Now let go. Keep your attention focused on your right hand. Observe what is happening without judging. Give yourself time to closely observe the entire area, and feel the relaxation that is growing. How does your hand feel now? Do you feel a difference?

5. Compare your right hand with your left hand. Experience how the muscle tone has become looser. Taking the time to feel the effects is more important than the performance of the exercise itself and should take significantly longer than the time of tensing and relaxing—about 30 seconds.

6. Continue with the exercise by consciously tensing and then releasing other parts of your body—your arms, legs, feet, abdomen, buttocks, chest, face, etc.

What is good for the body can also bring relief to the soul. Edmund Jacobson, the founder of progressive muscle relaxation, discovered that people suffering from spiritual tensions, fears, stress, and insecurities had an elevated muscle tone. The recognition that physical and spiritual tensions occurred in synchrony with one another led Jacobson to develop focused physical relaxation in the cause of spiritual relaxation.

Whenever you feel angry, annoyed, sad, desperate, frustrated, inhibited, fearful, shy, or emotionally unwell, consciously contract one muscle, almost as much as you can without feeling pain. While doing this focus on the emotion that is present for you, allow it to become strong and stronger, and then let it go, at the same time that you relax the muscle. Do you feel a spiritual relaxation in addition to the physical one?

The Five Phases

During your practice you may have already noticed that the progressive muscle relaxation occurs in five phases.

- ▲ **Feeling:** Before tensing the muscles (for example the fist), you concentrate. How do the muscles feel?
- ▲ **Tensing:** You tense the muscles (for example the fist) strongly, but not to the point of pain.
- ▲ **Maintaining tension:** You slowly count to seven while maintaining the tension and focusing on the muscle group. You continue breathing normally while doing this (except for exercises with buttocks).
- ▲ **Letting go:** You suddenly and consciously relax the muscles.
- ▲ **Feeling:** You continue to keep your attention on the muscle group. For about 30 seconds you continue to observe what is happening there (warmth, relaxation, etc.), without judging the feelings. You can feel this relaxation like the sound following the striking of a gong. Move on to the next muscle group only when the relaxation process can no longer be felt. To get a sense of how long 30 seconds is, you can count to thirty, or take a moment before the exercise to practice with a timer.

Three Possible Exercise Positions

You can carry out progressive muscle relaxation almost anywhere and at any time.

- ▲ **Lying down:** Lie on your back with your arms at your sides and legs parallel to one another. Ideally, do this every day before falling asleep or getting up, or before a lingam massage.
- ▲ **Sitting:** Your back is straight and your legs are extended directly in front of you. Your arms are slightly bent. This is a good position for exercising at work or before a meal.
- ▲ **Standing up:** Stand with your legs shoulder width apart, your

knees slightly bent, and your arms at your side. Your head is straight and your gaze is fixed on a point straight ahead of you to help you maintain your balance. This can be done discreetly while waiting at train stations, airports, etc.

▲ *The Seventeen Steps*

Full body relaxation and full body orgasms are related in a specific way. For this reason, it is important to include the entire body in the regular practice of progressive muscle relaxation. This sounds like a lot of effort, but the so-called seventeen steps according to Bernstein and Borkovec make a very effective full-body relaxation possible in relatively few steps.[8]

You will note a pleasant difference in your sexuality, and in your experience of lingam massage, if you regularly practice the following exercise sequence and take a full thirty seconds after each step to feel its effects. If time is short, it is better to do fewer exercises than to skimp on the time spent feeling after each.

For each step, it is best to inhale slowly as you tense the muscles, and to exhale rather quickly as you release them. Breathe normally during the 30-second feeling time.

1. Make a fist with your right hand and tense your fist and forearm. Then relax and breathe normally for 30 seconds.
2. With your elbow bent, press your right upper arm tightly against your upper body, or if you are lying down, against the floor while tensing the upper arm. Then relax and breathe.
3. Make a fist with your left hand and tense the fist and forearm. Then relax and breathe.
4. With your elbow bent, press your left upper arm tightly against your upper body, or if you are lying down, against the floor while tensing the upper arm. Then relax and breathe.
5. Raise your eyebrows as far as possible and tense your forehead. Then relax and breathe.

6. Wrinkle your nose, squint your eyes, and tense the upper part of your cheeks and nose. Then relax and breathe.

7. Press your teeth together (avoiding too much tension), pull the edges of your mouth back, and tense the lower cheeks and jaw. You can either press your tongue against your gums or leave it loosely in your mouth. Then relax and breathe.

8. Press your chin to your chest. Keep your spine straight and extend the muscles at the back of your neck as you contract the muscles at the front of your neck. In the mirror you will notice the formation of a double chin. Then relax and breathe.

During steps 9 to 11 you can hold your breath or keep breathing normally, as you prefer.

9. Try to bring your shoulder blades together on your back, then pull both shoulders forward. Then relax and breathe.

10. Pull your stomach in, as if you were trying to touch your spine with your belly button. Alternatively, push your stomach outward, like a Chinese Buddha figure. Or simply tense your stomach and make it hard as a board. While doing so, feel the tension in your abdominal muscles. Then relax and breathe.

11. Tense your buttocks and pelvis muscles as much as possible. Imagine pulling your internal organs up into your stomach. Squeeze your butt cheeks together and feel the tension in the muscles of the buttocks and pelvis. Then relax and breathe. (Continue repeating this exercise, especially while sitting down—this is very helpful for the circulation in the pelvic floor and thus for your potency!)

12. Simultaneously press the back of your right knee and thigh against the floor and feel the muscles on the front of your thigh. Then relax and breathe.

13. Lift the ball of your right foot up while keeping your heel on the ground. Pull the toes toward your head, stretching the foot. Feel the tension in your calf and foot. Then relax and breathe.

14. Stretch out the toes of your right foot as if they were claws. Proceed slowly to avoid cramps, then relax and breathe. If you do experience cramps, repeat step 13, since this relaxes the foot.
15. Simultaneously press the back of your left knee and thigh against the floor and feel the muscles of your thigh. Then relax and breathe.
16. Lift the ball of your left foot up while keeping your heel on the ground. Pull your toes toward your head, stretching the foot. Feel the tension in your calf and foot. Then relax and breathe.
17. Stretch out the toes of your left foot as if they were claws. Proceed slowly to avoid cramps, then relax and breathe. If you do experience cramps, repeat step 16, since this relaxes the foot.

As an addition, tense your anus, then relax and breathe. Many people experience tension or even pain during defecation, or else they have no muscle tone here at all. If you include the anus as an eighteenth step in this exercise, you will see how your growing consciousness of this region can help to resolve anal blockages and foster a new enthusiasm for life.

Conclusion: Stretch yourself and consciously return to the here and now!

The whole thing sounds more complicated than it is. The sequence is logical and, after you have read it a few times, easily recalled: right fist, right arm, left fist, left arm, tense the forehead, tense the lower cheeks, neck, shoulder blades, stomach, pelvis, right thigh, right calf, right toes, left thigh, left calf, left toes, anus, stretching, done.

To achieve an optimal effect, practice the seventeen steps daily for about four weeks, for example before getting up or going to bed. This will only take a few minutes, but you will see how your consciousness becomes more receptive day by day to sensory stimuli. If time is tight, you can focus on a single muscle group, as long as you continue to allow time afterward for deep feeling.

If you work at a desk, make a point of practicing the relaxation of your back. Pay special attention to your pelvis and buttocks. Your sexual energies are strongly dependent on how well you can relax these areas. Otherwise, simply focus on the muscle group that is the most tense.

Once you are comfortable with the exercise and quite accustomed to it, you can also begin to simply visualize the individual steps (for example while waiting for the bus, at the movies, etc.). This will work too, since muscles can learn and are able to "recall" the experience of tension and relaxation.

If you practice this exercise on a regular basis, after a few weeks you will be able to relax very quickly whenever you want to. This will be enormously helpful in allowing you to consciously enjoy a lingam massage. You will then also be optimally prepared to experience the Big Draw.

The Big Draw—The Theory

Many men are used to finishing their sexual experience with an ejaculation and thus going directly from arousal to deep relaxation. While this is a good way of doing things, the Big Draw is an interesting alternative to ejaculation and worth trying at least once.

During the male orgasm, the body prepares to put new life into the world. For that reason, all male organs and glands contribute their best minerals, trace elements, vitamins, and amino acids to the ejaculatory fluids. At the time of orgasm, the whole body is charged with extremely high bioelectric energy. According to Chinese medicine, sexual strength—called *ching*—is also given to the sperm. Ching is a very powerful source of energy but one that can only be used when it is "heated up," that is, when the body is in a state of sexual arousal. That, however, is also the time when the urge to ejaculate is at its strongest, meaning that the powerful energy leaves the body. While this may be a welcome relief and reduction of tension—especially for young men— and thus a net win for the body, many older men discover that frequent ejaculation makes them tired and weak, causing them to look for an alternative to ejaculation.

Taoist principles maintain that sexual energy can also be used to charge the male body with vitality and energy, and even to accelerate a man's spiritual development and "enlightenment." That is because the ching built up in sexual arousal is very valuable; men who make use of their sexual energy for their own benefit will be notably stronger than those who don't.

Stories tell of the legendary Yellow Emperor Huang Di, who ruled in about the twenty-sixth century BCE, who was said to have regularly transformed his ching for his own body's use. This practice was said to have rendered him nearly undefeatable. Other stories tell of later rulers who regularly visited a massage temple to receive erotic massage in connection with a repression of ejaculation to strengthen their male attributes. The Big Draw is thus not a new idea, but rather a rediscovery of ancient knowledge. The only new thing is the connection of the Big Draw with progressive muscle relaxation.

The Big Draw described in this book was discovered by Joseph Kramer when he was giving a lingam massage to breathing therapist Valnn Dayne, who at the end of the massage took about fifty strong breaths, then stopped breathing, contracted all the muscles of his body, and pulled up his feet and head. He remained in this position for about thirty seconds before exhaling and relaxing in deep joy.

▲ The Big Draw—The Technique

There is a Big Draw especially for men that recognizes their particularly fiery ching energy. As taught by Joseph Kramer, it is helpful if you first try the Big Draw without stimulation of the genitals.

1. Lie on your back and relax.
2. Practice rhythmic full breathing for about thirty minutes (see page 98), allowing your body to build up sufficient energy.* If you wish, move your pelvis and your whole body in rhythm with your breathing.

---

*If you like, you can listen to the CD *Tempelgongs* by Michael Vetter as background music.

3. Once you feel that it is time to prepare for the Big Draw, take fifty very quick, deep, and strong breaths, without interruption.

4. Now exhale and inhale as deeply as possible three times. After your third inhalation, hold your breath and contract all the muscles in your body, with strength but without pain, just as in progressive muscle relaxation. Pay special attention to contracting the PC muscle, the buttocks muscles, and the anus (this is the so-called anal lock). Lift your head slightly and pull your legs up to your chest. This is important for opening the neck and pelvis and allowing the free flow of energy.

5. Continue holding your breath in this position, and continue contracting your muscles until you feel that you won't be able to hold out much longer. (For beginners it is best to start with holding the breath for ten to twenty seconds, and not contracting the muscles too much.)

6. Then suddenly let go of all contractions, fall back onto your back, and return your breathing to the control of the autonomous nervous system. Give up all control.

7. Fully give in to what you feel, all the small and big sensations. Give in to your deep trust in the process, to the quiet, to the larger thing that is working within you at this moment, to letting go of the small, blinkered I. Perhaps like a wave that gives itself to the ocean. If emotions surface, whether quiet or strong, welcome and enjoy them.

8. Enjoy the relaxation. You will now experience your body returning by itself to its normal state. Perhaps you will even notice that your mind, after its "flight of the phoenix," is getting ready to return to your body, perhaps in deeper connection with it than before. What remains is peace and the memory of the depth of the experience.

If, as the giving partner of a lingam massage, you are directing and accompanying your partner in a Big Draw, it is important not to touch him or speak with him afterward, since his energy system is very sensitive at this moment. If possible, cover your partner with a cloth to make sure he feels protected. But nothing more! Sit down quietly or leave the room for about ten minutes to allow your partner to gradually return from his experience to reality.

Men's Experiences with the Big Draw

- ▲ I unexpectedly found solutions for the problems in my life, suddenly everything became clear.
- ▲ I saw myself from a great height and was able to observe my life from a "higher" perspective.
- ▲ I felt a deep peace, a kind of recognition or spiritual awakening, I felt like both laughing and crying, and did both.
- ▲ I felt joy, happiness, peace, contentedness.
- ▲ My consciousness increased rapidly and I felt gold-white light come through me as if I was standing in the center of a great sun.
- ▲ I felt as if my consciousness had left my skull, and it was wonderful to be free of the limitations of my body for a few moments. Then after a few moments I experienced the reentry into my body—I felt fresh, new, cleansed, regenerated.
- ▲ During breathing I felt my power animal, the eagle. When I let go after the Big Draw, it was as if the eagle was taking me under its wings and carrying me into the air.
- ▲ After the Big Draw I felt a great strength, as if I could have torn up trees. The next morning I woke early and felt in great shape, it was as if the Big Draw had reduced my need for sleep.
- ▲ In the days after my Big Draw I was able to work and accomplish more than I had in the weeks before.
- ▲ When I tried the Big Draw for the first time, this wonderful feeling lasted for half an hour. With continuing practice I have experienced it lasting for several days and even weeks.

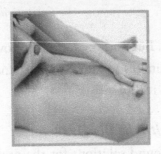

3
The Lingam
and Prostate Massage

Sex is completely innocent energy.
Sex is life, pulsing within you,
Existence, vibrating within you.
Do not cripple this energy.
Rather, allow it to come to the highest flower
Of its expression.
In this, sex becomes love.

—OSHO

A CONSCIOUS APPROACH
TO LINGAM MASSAGE

In the previous chapters, we explored the various components of the lingam massage in detail. This chapter shows you how to integrate those components into a smooth and flowing massage.

Notes for the Massage Giver
You are now the active partner: part of your job is to take charge so that your partner can fully trust you and give in to his experience. Lovingly

prepare a space for the massage—a clean room, clean sheets on the floor, and protection from interruptions are all necessary. You can also add relaxing music, scents, flowers, and so forth, if you like.

Prepare a clear framework for the massage. Ideally, you will have already agreed on a timeframe within which you are there for your partner's needs only. Be ready to open your own channels to arousal, and to be sensitive to the wishes and possibilities of your partner, but be clear with yourself that this is his journey. If you experience your own needs during the massage, take note of them lovingly, but consciously put them aside and promise yourself to look after them as soon as you have your own opportunity. While you are giving a lingam massage, your needs remain clearly in the background, unless you feel that for physical or psychological reasons, you are not able to continue the massage as agreed. Do not be disappointed if the massage does not go as you had hoped. Again, it is your partner's journey and he has the space to express himself sexually as he wishes, as long as this doesn't go beyond your limits.

If your partner does not get an erection, this doesn't mean that he is not enjoying the massage; there are many reasons why a man may not have an erection. But it may also be the case that your touch is not the right one at that moment. Ask him whether the way you are touching him is good for him! If you are unsure during the massage, it is always helpful to ask short and simple questions that your partner can answer with a nod or shake of the head or with one or two words: "Is it pleasant for you, if I do . . . , or would you like to be touched differently?" "Is the pressure good like this?" "What do you need right now?" Asking questions also reassures your partner that you are taking his feelings into account. However, the degree to which a verbal exchange makes sense differs depending on the person. Here too, follow the wishes of your partner.

If your partner does not get an erection, you have to take this into account during the course of the massage. This means a focus on gentle and soft touch. For example, you will need to use a gentle and slow touch on the foreskin, and gently massage the spot under the glans. It is especially important that the lingam is touched with a great degree of feeling. Do not try to "force" an erection. This will not work and is completely unimportant for the lingam massage.

If your partner signals you that he is close to ejaculating, stop or slow down your touch. Stroke the entire body and breathe with your partner. Encourage your partner to focus on breathing deeply and using his PC pump (see page 37). You can also place your hands under his pelvis and make gentle, swinging movements with him. This will automatically encourage him to breathe deeply into his pelvis and relax.

If he comes very close to ejaculation, you can use one hand to gently pull his testicles away from his body, while using the middle finger of your other hand to press down on the "point of a million pieces of gold" on the perineum directly behind the lingam root. In doing so you close off the urethra at the lower end of the prostate. If you do this, the semen can no longer be pushed out of the lingam, and the urge to ejaculate will decrease.

Once the arousal curve has lowered, resume the lingam massage. If possible, accompany your partner during the waves of this journey. Continue allowing the waves to rise, and continue to distribute the energy around his body before he ejaculates. This allows your Shiva to experience several small or larger orgasms without ejaculation during a lingam massage. But always remember to take it with humor and calm if not everything goes as planned. Even in real life a surfer will need some experience before he can ride the waves.

If an ejaculation should occur after a few minutes, then enjoy and celebrate it; the next time your partner may last a little longer. It is an unsubstantiated prejudice that an ejaculation spells the end of enjoyment. Many men are able to continue receiving a lingam massage after a brief rest, although some others may experience further touch as uncomfortable at this stage. Speak about this with your partner and either end the massage or celebrate it again after an appropriate pause.

After the massage, take enough time to talk about what you experienced. When the interaction is completely finished and you have energetically separated from your partner, look well after yourself and your own needs.

Notes for the Massage Recipient

You deserve it! It is your time to do nothing, not to perform. You don't have to live up to any expectations. You can ejaculate when you want, or not at all. You may have an erection or not. You can sigh and moan loudly, or enjoy in silence. You can be horny, sad, angry, or fearful. You can laugh and cry. Everything is allowed, as long as you respect the limits of your partner. This is your time—make the best of it!

In receiving a lingam massage you have the opportunity to discover entirely new aspects of your sexuality. Let go of old ideas about what sex should be. Let go of expectations that you feel obliged to fulfill. Continue breathing deeply, since your breathing will return your attention to your body. Try to breathe deeply during the entire massage. Breathe, feel yourself, take note of your sensations and thoughts, regardless of whether you are feeling aroused or simply pleasantly touched. Express your sexuality by making sounds or movements. Give clear signs to your partner. Express your likes and dislikes, tell him or her what you need to feel good, horny, comforted, aroused, or more deeply meditative. Also tell your partner what is unpleasant, what you would like to experience differently, and maybe how. Your partner cannot know everything unless you make it clear.

Let go of wondering whether you will have an erection or not, and focus on your inner sensations, as described in chapter 2, in the section on feeling your lingam (see page 90). Feel how the touches from your partner affect parts deep inside of you. Allow your whole being to be touched. Feel the various types of touch and be conscious and aware of their differences:

▲ How does it feel to be touched slowly and gently?
▲ How does it feel to be touched quickly and energetically?
▲ How does your lingam feel when it is stroked up and down?

▲ How do your glans, your shaft, your testicles, and perineum feel?

▲ Which touch do you like the most, which the least?

▲ How aroused are you?

▲ How deep is your breathing?

Be conscious of the progression of your arousal. Inhale and exhale deeply and feel how you can influence your arousal through your breathing. Notice also how you can focus your breathing on different parts of your body. Perhaps you will note that you can use your breathing and your PC muscles to lessen the urge to ejaculate, and increase the quality of sensation. If not, simply take note of this. Even if you are only feeling minimally aroused, it is good to take note of it, without judgment and without the feeling that there should be more. Love what you experience and relax within it.

Continue breathing deeply. Feel when it works for you to allow your arousal to decrease a bit when you're not yet ready to ejaculate. Give a clear signal to your partner so that he or she can stop touching your lingam and instead distribute the energy throughout your body. In rhythm with your breathing, pull the muscles of your pelvic floor together and relax them again. Try for yourself what feels better: contracting during inhalation and letting go during exhalation, or the other way around. Repeat this as often as you like. What is happening to your arousal? Where in your body are you feeling your sexual energy?

If you feel very aroused, visualize how your sexual energy is pulled upward as you inhale—along your spine to the top of your head. As you exhale, feel it flow down along the center of the front of your body, back to the perineum. Allow your sexual energy to flow and spread throughout your body. Playfully use your PC and pelvic muscles, sometimes quickly, sometimes slowly, as if you were squeezing juice out of a ripe lemon. Experience how the energy "arrives" at the top of your body.

Perhaps it is possible for you to expand your arousal a great deal, causing the muscles in your body to feel a warm orgasmic feeling, without ejaculation. This kind of orgasm implodes within your body and extends upward, rather than exploding downward and out of your body in ejaculation.

Whatever happens, approach the experience playfully. Don't stress yourself. If the ejaculation comes sooner than you had intended, enjoy it wholeheartedly. Do not try to stop an ejaculation that is already happening. It would be a shame to miss the feeling of warmth that an orgasm can provide. Perhaps you want to take a short break before continuing to enjoy the lingam massage. Or perhaps you have had enough and you simply want to be taken into your partner's arms and held. Simply feel within yourself and express your needs.

If your lingam massage was not ended prematurely by an ejaculation, ask yourself what conclusion you want to the massage this time.

▲ Do you want the arousal to implode in your body without ejaculation? Ask your partner to use a technique that you particularly enjoy. Allow your arousal to spread throughout your body while you remain relaxed. You do not have to go to extremes—a 60.percent arousal level is fine and can be very harmonizing, although you can also go to 90.percent or 95 percent if you know how to do it without getting stressed, or going too far. At some point give your partner the clear signal that he or she should end the massage and stop touching you. Now practice the Big Draw. Feel the energy in your body, and remain present in the here and now.

▲ Would you prefer a calm, meditative, and gentle conclusion? Would you prefer not to ejaculate, not to practice a Big Draw, but just to breathe calmly and let the massage finish gently? This too is possible and can be very energizing. If so, give your partner a clear sign that he or she should slowly end the massage. Be clear about what you need now; perhaps you want to be held, or just left alone.

▲ Do you want to allow your energy to explode in an ejaculation? Ask your partner to use a technique that you particularly enjoy and have an orgasm with ejaculation. Appreciate your orgasm and feel it for as long as possible. Here too, give clear signals about what you need now to be full and nourished.

After the massage, give yourself and your partner enough space to talk about what you experienced.

The Energetic Sequence of a Lingam Massage

Men's sexuality and women's sexuality have more in common than we think. Because the sexual organs of both sexes develop from the same embryonic parts, there are many physical and emotional similarities. For example, women experience stimulation of the clitoris in much the same way that men experience massage on the areas to the right and left of the frenulum, and on the back edge of the glans. Women's sensations during G-spot stimulation are similar to men's sensations during prostate massage.

However, the sexuality of men and women is fundamentally different on an energetic level, in the way that sexual expression is lived and transformed. Women have a more receptive sexual nature. A woman opens herself, allows entry, and receives energy in the form of the lingam and male semen. Men, in contrast, carry their sexual organs on the outside: they rise, penetrate, and give their energy to the outside. This is a very different way of moving through life and experiencing sexuality. Men thus encounter sexuality with decisiveness, clarity, and directness, which is different than a woman's approach.

Clarity, potency, and goal-orientation are characteristically male qualities. They are symbolized by a powerful erection that wants to be lived and celebrated. In lingam massage, men experience how they can consciously develop these qualities in their sexuality and anchor them within their hearts and minds. Men experience softness, devotion, and openness primarily via anal or prostate massage, which will be discussed in more detail in the next chapter.

Energetically, a lingam massage proceeds in a fundamentally different way than a yoni massage, which is why the approach and execution are also very different. The lingam massage is thus primarily (but not exclusively) characterized by strength and energy, while the mood during a yoni massage is more (but not entirely) emotional and fluid.

Energy proceeds in waves during lingam massage, and the massage techniques are designed accordingly. After the genital region has been aroused and the root has been brought to flower (see page 138), a lot of energy is built up relatively quickly in a sequence of repeating phases. This is followed by massage techniques to hold this energy, stroke it, and distribute it throughout the body. These techniques offer men the possibility of adding durability to the quickly achieved arousal, and of experiencing climaxes or orgasms several times. Chinese teachings refer to bringing the essential energy, or ching, which is located at the lower end of the spine, upward along the spine using breathing and massage techniques, and distributing it throughout the body. This refines the ching into a purified essence that nourishes the body and expands consciousness.

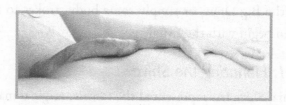

THE LINGAM MASSAGE—
PHASE BY PHASE

Before beginning the massage, both partners should take enough time to talk about what is going to take place. Talk about your expectations, wishes, fears, and needs, and be as honest as possible. If you will be receiving a lingam massage, you may wish to speak about how your lingam feels today and what needs you are having. It is good for the receiving partner to articulate changes he may wish to make in his life. We often see that the energy that is released through orgasm or the Big Draw supports the consciousness of the recipient to bring about decisive positive change in many aspects of his life.

If you will be giving a lingam massage, you can ask your partner the following questions, especially if you know each other: "What would you like to experience over the next ninety minutes? Is there a change that you would like to experience as a result of the lingam massage?"

Listen carefully and be conscious of the fact that nothing that is said has to do with you personally. If you like, speak about your own fears. Make sure not to judge anything that is being said. Explain to your partner the sequence of the coming massage. Introduce him to the breathing rhythm and explain to him that it is helpful to breathe deeply and consciously during the massage.

Talk about whether your partner would prefer to have an orgasm without ejaculation, try a Big Draw, or whether he would like to experience an orgasm with ejaculation. This discussion doesn't mean that he can't change his mind during the massage. Agree on clear signs, so the recipient can indicate when he is approaching ejaculation whether or not he wants to ejaculate at that time, or whether he needs room to practice the Big Draw, or simply some body strokes to redirect his energy. Then begin with the ritual.

▲ Phase 1: Honoring the Shiva

For millennia, Shiva has represented the tantric, original male strength. The first phase of lingam massage is about honoring the man—a representation of Shiva—in his whole beauty, naturalness, and especially in his masculinity as carrier of the lingam. Careful preparation of the massage space and a loving initial dialogue are especially important for men, who are all too often expected to "get straight to the point" of things, rather than respond to a gentle introduction.

Underneath the tough shell of many men is often a sensitive and emotional being. This more emotional part usually remains hidden because men, unlike women, do not have centuries of experience in dealing with their feelings. Ideally, the heart of a man can be expressed in his sexuality and represented by his lingam. If a man attempts to separate his heart from his sexual life, he will inevitably end up denying his heart. Knowing this, we try to reconnect heart and sexuality in lingam massage; that process begins with honoring the man and his lingam.

The following honoring ritual helps you to see in each male lingam the shining creative potential of love as it manifests on Earth. It also provides ways of honoring this creative potential as a source of happiness and well-being. This ritual allows you to open a door, on the other side of which a man can choose to let go of his fears and performance thinking, and reveal his heart to you in love.

▪ Preparations

As the giving partner, prepare a loving, pleasant, and warm space (at least 80 degrees Farenheit) with nice fabrics, flowers, candles, and sensual background music. In the center of the room, prepare the massage area. Have all the tools handy that you may need for the massage (for example feathers, fans, cloths, furs, massage oil, lubricants,* a bowl of hot water, wash cloth, and a small stove). Both of you should wear a nice kimono, a sarong, or a sensual bathrobe.

As the giving partner, take charge of the massage session. Sit down on the prepared massage area facing one another. It is your job to clearly tell your partner what he should do. Avoid sentences like "maybe you could . . ." or "would you please . . . ," since these are unclear and lead people to think. Make sure that you truly mean every sentence that you say.

1. As giver, sit in front of your partner and look at him as if seeing him for the very first time. Hold your left hand out to him with the palm facing upward and say, "Please give me your hand." The receiver places his right hand with the palm facing downward into yours. Then say, "Now I give you my hand," while giving him your right hand with the palm facing down. He places his left palm under it, so that he is carrying your hand in his. In this way you form a

---

*We recommend the lubricant by Pjur (www.pjur.com) since it remains smooth even during an extended massage and does not get sticky.

circle of give and take. This is important since even though you are the only one giving a massage, it is impossible to touch someone without being touched yourself.

Feel your breathing and breathe in the same rhythm as your partner. Deepen your breathing. Take in the character of your partner. Keep your gaze on him, open and friendly. Create an internal readiness to touch and allow yourself to be touched. Make sure not to let your gaze become too fixed.

2. Now offer a personal invitation, for example: "I invite you on a sensual journey to the center of your masculinity, and will do my best to ensure that you can fully trust me and give in to what is happening. For the duration of the massage I will be there for you only, and for everything that you need. When you are ready for the massage, pull your hands back very slowly."

3. Now bless your partner's three main chakras. With a special oil touch his pubic mound and say, "May your desire and masculinity

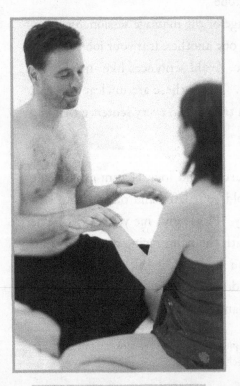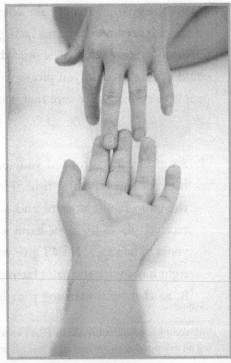

Phase 1: Honoring the Shiva

flower with strength." Then again take a little oil and touch his heart, saying, "May your heart open up and shine for everyone." Finally, take a little more oil and place it on his forehead as you say, "May your desire expand your vision and understanding."

4. Sit down close behind your partner. Place your right hand on his lower abdomen and your left hand on his heart. (At this point your right hand can begin to lightly touch and honor his lingam from the top if this is all right for him.) Lightly pull your partner toward you so that he can lean against you as if on a chair with a backrest. Make sure that he lets his head rest against your shoulder by gently and tenderly pulling him toward you. Now hold him and gently rock him. If you like, you can also hum a song at this point. Take a part of his tension and allow him to become a bit heavier against you, until he lets go completely and is letting himself be carried and held by you. Breathe in rhythm with him and deepen this breathing.

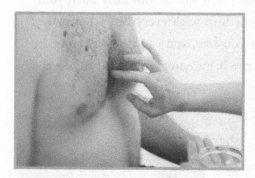

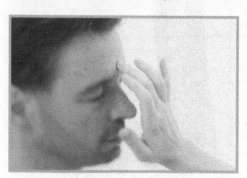

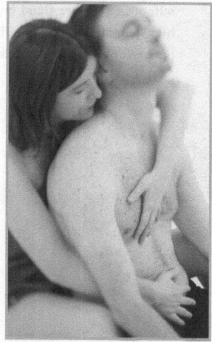

Phase 1: Honoring the Shiva

5. Straighten your partner's back. Gently play with the hair on the back of his head, massage his scalp and gently and sensually tug on his hair. Even if your partner has little or no hair, it is good to at least visualize playing with his hair, since energetically speaking, all of us have hair.

6. Now stand in front of your partner and say, "Please stand in front of me." Use your hands to show him precisely where you want him to stand. Then begin drawing tantric strands of joy around him. Tenderly touch his left cheek with your right hand and make a counter-clock wise spiral from the top of his body to the bottom using your palm, until your hands reach his feet. Symbolically, this gesture connects the sky with the earth. A counter-clockwise spiral unites the spiritual with the physical. While drawing these strands, say to your partner: "You don't need to do anything anymore. Just observe, breathe, and let yourself be taken care of. I am spinning a strand of happiness around you."

7. Place your hands on his feet and bow down. Inwardly open yourself: open your heart and honor him with everything that makes him recognizable as a man. If you like, you can now say an inner prayer, for example the Sanskrit: "Om namah Shiva—I honor the godly inside you."

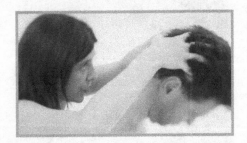
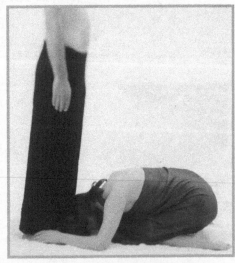

Phase 1: Honoring the Shiva

8. It is now time to disrobe your partner. Slowly undo the belt of his kimono or the knot of his sarong. Celebrate this slowly and with joy, taking pleasure from each touch and gesture. Now gently run your fingers under the material and slowly glide the kimono across his shoulders or the sarong off his body. Stand behind your partner and let the fabric slide down along his back. Play with this for a while by making the most of the sensation of fabric on skin. Then carefully and neatly place the kimono or sarong off to the side.

9. Now touch your partner by marking the energy cycle of his body. Beginning at the coccyx, stroke his spine from bottom to top (the Governor vessel) and repeat this two or three times, using a gentle touch that you can also accompany with a warm breath. Touching

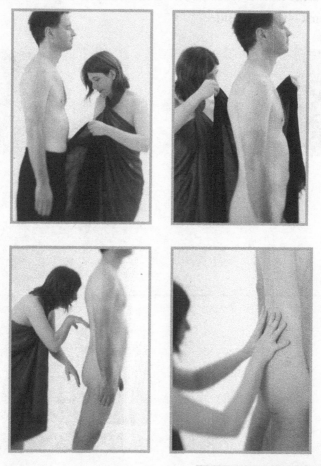

Phase 1: Honoring the Shiva

the neck can be especially pleasant, and will often cause a slight shudder. Then use your flat hands to stroke from the head along the back and the outside of the legs until you reach his feet. Stroke the feet and proceed upward along the insides of the legs, across the loins, the stomach, the center of the chest, and down along the inside of the arms to the palms. From there, run along the backs of the hands and arms, to the throat, face, head, and down again along the back across the outside of the legs to the feet. Stroke the feet and continue as described above. Repeat this about three times.

10. From behind, slowly press against his body and again place your right hand on his lower abdomen and your left hand on his heart. Speak gently into his ear: "Please lie down on your stomach, with your arms next to your body." With this you begin the massage of his back—the yang side.

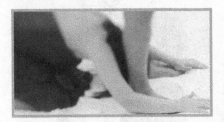
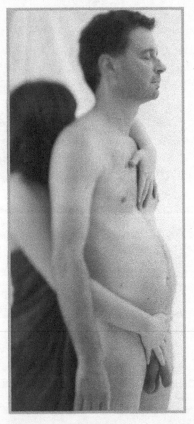

Phase 1: Honoring the Shiva

▲ Phase 2: The Preparatory Full-Body Massage

After the honoring of Shiva, the second phase is a full-body massage that sets the stage for lingam massage. To touch and massage the body is to honor it. In this massage, it is less important to carry out every step as described here, and more important to begin a dialogue with your hands and the body of the recipient. It is not technique that you use for the touch, but your love, your undivided attention, and your joy in what you are doing. Open the man: touch, knead, rock, and stroke him so that he feels completely accepted and loved. This will allow his body to become more receptive to the sensual and arousing pleasures for which this massage is a preparation.

Since this is a sensual massage, it is wonderful to create an erotic and sexual atmosphere from beginning to end. Do not avoid the genital area, but rather continue touching it during the massage to create a gentle opening even before the genital massage. Breathing during this phase is calm and deep; it should go deep down into the pelvis. You may choose to use the following during your massage: a feather, a small fur, massage oil, three washcloths, a bowl with hot water, a small hotplate.

▪ Massaging the Yang Side

1. Your partner is lying on his stomach. Sit behind your partner's head and undress yourself as slowly and sensually as you earlier undressed him. Take your sarong or another nice fabric and gently place it over your partner's head. Move to his feet and from there pull the fabric across his back, making small waves while doing so. Slowly and steadily pull the fabric off across his feet.

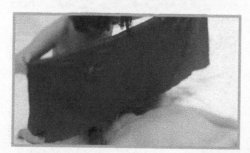 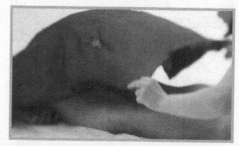

Phase 2: The Preparatory Full-Body Massage

2. With a feather, touch your partner's entire back with long, feeling strokes. Alternate between quick, teasing strokes and long, relaxed ones. Make sure to touch the entire body evenly. For variety you can turn the feather around and use the stem to lightly prick his back, or you can use furs, your hair, or any kind of erotic accessories in this game of the senses.

3. Use your fingertips to touch his entire body. Here too you can alternate between very slow and slightly faster movements to create erotic tension. The important thing is that you also enjoy the touch, a feeling that will then naturally transfer on to your Shiva.

4. Pour a little oil into your hand and distribute it gently in regular long strokes across the entire body. Base oils like almond, sesame, or jojoba oil are best suited for this, or other natural oils for professional massage. Let the oil flow into your hand before placing it on your partner's back. Let your hands flow like waves and glide them steadily across your partner's body. Make sure to keep your wrists loose so that your hands touch the skin in a soft and gentle way.

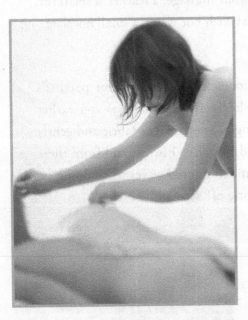
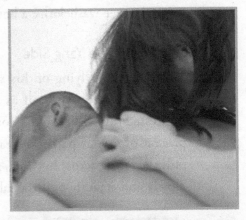
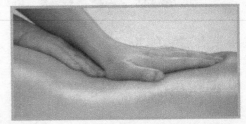

Phase 2

5. Sit down near your partner's head and massage both sides of his back one after another, using circling movements from head to buttocks, in each case moving away from the spine. Glide your hands upward along the outside of the body with gently swinging movements. You can also use the tips of your index, middle, and ring fingers and massage both halves of the back deeply and simultaneously in small, quick circles. Also massage his shoulders and neck.

6. Sit on your partner's right side and massage his right arm from the shoulder, across the top of his arm to his palm, with flowing and kneading movements. Repeat the same thing on your partner's left side with his left arm.

7. Now massage your partner's right leg from the hip to the foot. Visualize being in a tender but sometimes strong wave that envelops the whole leg, presses against it, and then flows back. Repeat the same with the left leg.

8. Now sit between your partner's legs, take him by the hip joints and gently rock his entire pelvis back and forth.

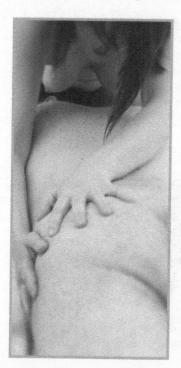
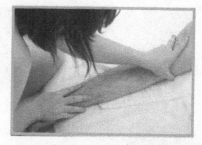
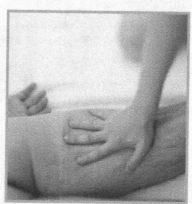

Phase 2

9. Begin touching his buttocks rhythmically and strongly using your fingertips, starting with one buttock and then moving to the other. Then work both buttocks like a drum (again one after the other), using the edges of your hands, drumming rhythmically and deeply into the tissue. Again make sure that these movements flow easily from your wrists. Conclude by making a small fist and tapping the coccyx region. This awakens your partner's kundalini energy, which you then direct up from the coccyx along the spine to the top of his head, using your thumbs.

10. Now strongly knead both your partner's buttocks one after another, with the goal of warming them up. Always proceed from the inside upward and outward.

11. Now blow gentle hot breaths onto your partner's skin. Start with one or two spots on the coccyx, then move upward along his spine. When your breath reaches the back of his neck, gently and sensually lie down on your partner's back. Use this to create a small break for yourself. Breathe in synchrony with your partner, and then sit beside

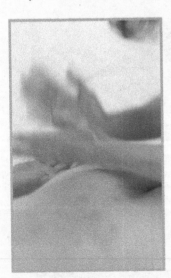
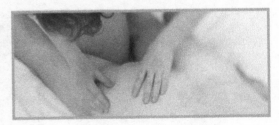
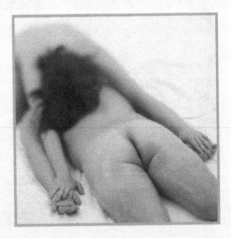

him again. Stroke the entire back of his body from top to bottom and rest for a short while at the soles of his feet. Stroke the feet and create a sensual transition before coming back to a rest at his head. Place your face on his back, press your hands against his, and remain lying there for a little while. Then say to him, "Please turn over."

▪ Massaging the Yin Side

1. Your partner is lying on his back. Touch and stroke the entire front of your partner using a feather, a fur, your hair, or anything else that is suitable, just as you did on his back.
2. Then use your fingertips to massage the yin side as you did the yang side, following the same guidelines as in step 3 above (see page 128).
3. Begin with an "erotic washing." Being washed from head to foot is a sensual pleasure like a warm embrace. Such a cleansing should be understood holistically, since it also frees the soul from emotional baggage. For this cleansing, prepare a bowl with warm to hot water before the massage and place it on a small hotplate where it can be easily reached. Also place three washcloths nearby. You can mix a few drops of a nice essential oil in the water to create a pleasant smell during the cleansing.

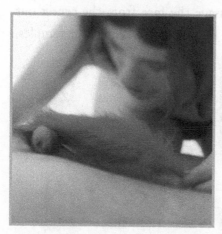
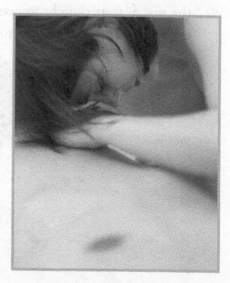

Place a warm washcloth over your partner's heart and apply gentle pressure. Then place another, less hot, washcloth on the lingam. Now apply light pressure on his heart area with one hand and on his lingam with your other hand. Continue breathing in the same rhythm as your partner.

Prepare a third washcloth and place this one on your partner's forehead. Here, too, apply gentle pressure. Now take the washcloth away from the forehead, dip it again into hot water, and begin lovingly washing the front of your partner's body, gently and sensually.

Conclude by taking all cloths from the body and using your hands to rub your partner's body dry to make sure he doesn't get cold.

4. Sit down again at your partner's head and begin a facial massage. Place a few drops of a scented oil (base oil with a few drops of good essential oil, such as ylang ylang, orange, rose, or jasmine) in your hand. Let your Shiva smell the oil and then gently distribute it across his face, making sure not to get any oil into his eyes. Continue using your lightly oiled hands to stroke very gently from the center of the face across each side toward the ears. Then use the tips of your thumbs to massage the face from the center out to the ears, and from the top to the bottom. Massage the temples,

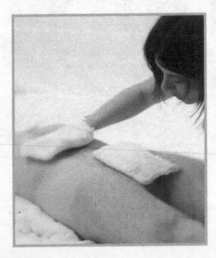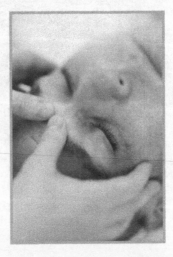

Phase 2

the nose, and the lips, letting your touch gently fade away behind the ears.

5. Pour oil into your hand and distribute it across your partner's chest and stomach. Sit down close to your partner's head to make this easier for you.

6. Massage your partner's front by stroking down along the center of his body from the throat to the pubic mound, and then returning to the top along the edge of his body via the armpits, shoulders, neck, and head.

7. Sit on your partner's left side and massage his chest by drawing a circle around his heart from the center upward and outward. Begin with the right breast before moving on to the left.

8. Very gently massage his belly in a clockwise direction (the natural flow of digestion). You can support your partner's back during this belly massage by sliding your right hand under his lower back. This will help him to relax and enjoy the massage.

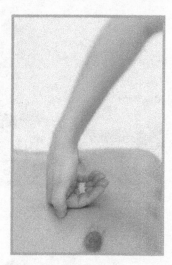
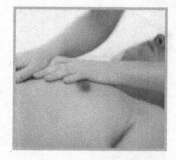
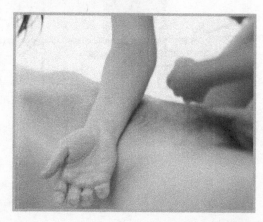

Phase 2

9. Massage first his left and then his right leg from the hip to the foot, as described above in step #7 for the yang side (see page 129).

10. Sit at your partner's feet. Hold both feet by the heels and pull lightly on your partner's legs, creating a slight tension. Use your hold on his legs to rock him gently back and forth.

11. Now place the soles of his feet against your belly. Inhale and exhale deeply, allowing your partner to feel with his feet how your belly expands and contracts.

12. Slowly draw your partner's legs far enough apart to give you plenty of room to begin the lingam massage. Be very attentive as you do this; by opening the legs you are also opening the innermost part of your partner. This opening should never go beyond his limits, so it is very important to take even the smallest resistance seriously.

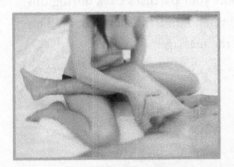

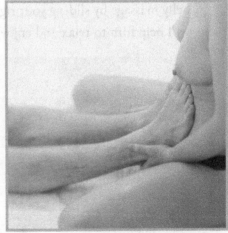

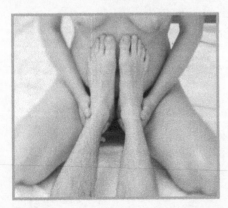

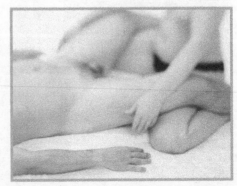

▲ Phase 3: Awakening Desire

The third phase is called "Awakening Desire." It prepares a man for genital massage by gradually and playfully approaching his lingam. This transition time is important, as it enables a man to give in to his sensations calmly and without expectations. You can include in this massage all the sensual areas of the body—including the neck, chest, face, the area between the legs (but not the lingam), the fingers and toes. Stimulate the areas around the lingam lovingly, without touching the lingam directly. Playfully tug on the lingam hair. In this phase, the recipient's breathing will tend to be rather calm, though it may speed up at times. It is important to remind your partner to breathe deeply into his pelvis.

When you are receiving a lingam massage, you can enjoy this loving and attentive touch and let go of all expectations. Receive, breathe, and follow any impulses to move your body that may come with the pleasurable sensations.

1. **Heart-genital touch:** Rub your hands together until they are hot, then place your left hand on your partner's heart and your right hand on his lingam. Be fully present and feel your healing energy nourishing his heart and lingam. Then massage the area between

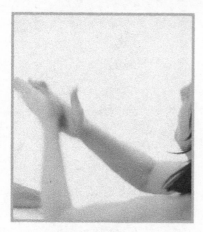
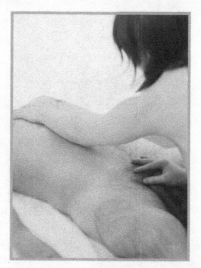

Phase 3: Awakening Desire

the two places: use your left hand to very slowly stroke along the midline from the heart down to the lingam. In this way you are creating a connection for your partner between his heart and his sexuality. This connection is the focus of lingam massage, and helps to charge the second and fourth chakras.

2. **Everything in hand:** Place your hands on your partner's knees and use both hands to stroke from his knees along the insides of his thighs, up to the inguinal groove—the indentation between the legs and the genitals. Repeat this stroke three to four times. Then hold the genitals with gentle pressure by making a ring around the root of the penis and the testicles. Gently pulsate your fingers in rhythm with your partner's breathing, and slightly faster.

3. **Cross-stroke:** Place your hands on your partner's knees, with your left hand resting on his right knee and your right hand on his left knee. Now begin to move your left hand with gentle strokes—from the right knee across the lingam to your partner's left breast. Once your left hand has reached his lingam, begin a similar diagonal movement with your right hand from the left knee across the lingam to the right breast. When your right hand has reached the

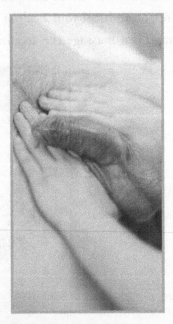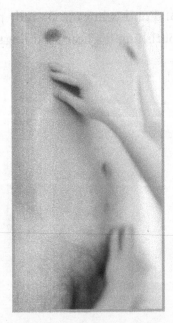

Phase 3

lingam, your left hand will be on your partner's left breast; bring your left hand back down to your partner's right knee as your right hand reaches reached your partner's right breast. In this stroke, the important thing is to make sure that with each motion, the lingam and the breast are lovingly caressed, awoken, and teased. This may sound somewhat complicated but is very easy in practice. You will quickly find a steady rhythm.

4. **Oil rub:** Lovingly apply oil to the entire lingam, remembering that anointing a partner with oil has been a special honoring ritual for millennia. Allow yourself plenty of time while doing this and include your partner's entire body. Use sufficient, but not too much oil since you will otherwise reduce the pleasurable friction on the lingam. I personally prefer a good lubricant, since oils quickly become thick and sticky.

5. **Lingam shiatsu:** Use your thumb and index finger to press the lingam from its base to its tip. Begin at the front and then move on to the sides. This awakens the inner tissue and stimulates the reflex zones of the lingam.

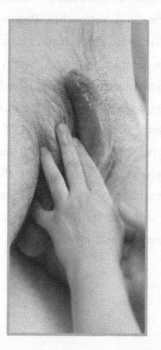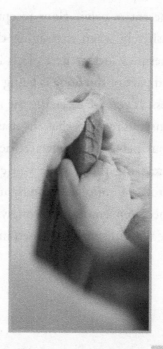

Phase 3

▲ Phase 4: From the Root to the Flower

Usually, stimulation of the male genitals is confined to the shaft and head of the lingam, while the root—the perineum and testicles—is given little or no attention at all. However, this region is very important for men, helping them to bring their sexuality to full flower. Massage of the perineum also stimulates the prostate from the outside. This helps your partner get in touch with or deepen his connection with the more passive and receptive side of his sexuality.

Moreover, an intensive massage in this area paves the way to a gentle and implosive (internally directed) orgasm, an enjoyable alternative to the explosive orgasm with ejaculation. On the perineum is the acupressure point *jen mo,* discussed earlier (see page 25), which in Taoism and sexual kung fu is called the "point of a million pieces of gold." It is located directly behind the penis root on a spot that feels very soft and flexible. Pressure on this spot causes energy to rise in the meridians that originate here; it is a sort of root for the whole body.

This phase is not about orgasm, but about awakening the area around the perineum and the testicles, to stimulate circulation and make the entire pelvic floor receptive and permeable. Proceed gently and sensitively when massaging this area, since unpleasant feelings can sometimes surface here. This is completely normal when a rather neglected part of the body is being sensitized and brought back to consciousness. If you are receiving the massage, focus your attention on the sensations and feelings that the massage of this area evokes. If you like, move your pelvis and contract the muscles of the pelvic floor as you inhale, relaxing them while you exhale. You can support the release of any stored emotions by loudly moaning as you exhale. Hearing you experience your emotions strongly will also motivate your partner to continue working with increased intensity and love.

Phase 4: From the Root to the Flower

1. **The big path:** Sit between your partner's legs, facing his lingam as it rests on his belly. Hold the lingam loosely with your right hand. Use your left hand (with your fingertips pointing toward the anus) to stroke from the anus along the perineum to the base of the testicles. Then turn your hand so that your fingertips are pointing toward the glans (head) of the lingam. Stroke between the testicles and along the underside of the shaft up to the tip of the lingam. This stroke helps to bring energy from the first chakra into the second chakra. Then use your whole hand to stroke down the lingam, across the testicles, and back to the perineum. For many men this is a very pleasurable experience. Repeat this three to five times.

2. **Scrotum massage:** Use your fingers to stroke along the testicles and spermatic cords. Gently touch the scrotum, feel each testicle, and take the spermatic cords between your fingers. Stretch the skin of the scrotum and massage it thoroughly.

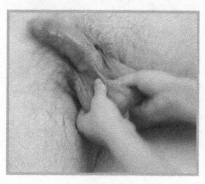

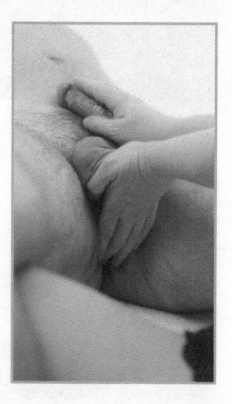

3. **Exploring the root:** Begin to explore the area between the anus and the testicles. Feel the mound behind the testicles that forms the root of the lingam. Place your hand on this root, press it extensively with circular movements. At the same time, you can also take the lingam root between your thumb and fingers to massage it. A good deal of pressure is often welcome at the lingam root.

4. **Massaging the prostate:** Follow the lingam root toward the anus and pay attention to the area at which your fingers encounter the soft and flexible *jen mo* point, behind which lies the prostate. The prostate feels like a small, solid, round rubber ball. Ask your partner whether this is the right spot and continue to have him give you feedback. You will probably find that you can press quite deeply

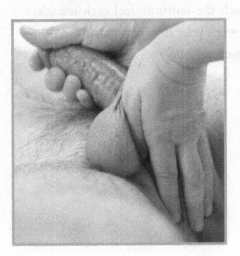
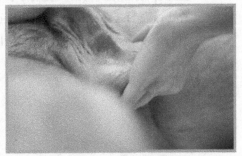
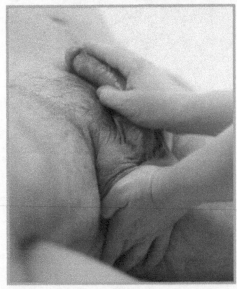

and strongly in this soft area. Massage it thoroughly with two or three fingers. You can also carry out a vibration massage by pressing your finger gently on the prostate and vibrating it. Vary your speed and pressure in a way that is pleasant for your partner. Ask him! Continue to gently include the lingam in this exercise. As we know, the massage of the prostate is only pleasurable if the lingam has already been awoken.

5. **Vibrating the root:** Make a fist and press your knuckles gently but steadily against the perineum. Then use your other hand to gently pull the scrotum upward, so that you can place your fist directly underneath it. Begin vibrating your fist. You can do this quite strongly and for a long time. If you are using your right hand to vibrate and massage the perineum, you can use your left hand to strongly massage the inside of the right thigh to the perineum. Then change hands—have your left fist massage the perineum, while your right hand massages the inside of the left thigh.

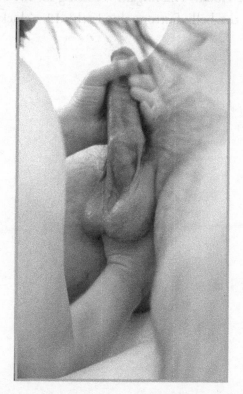

▲ *Phase 5: Awakening the Lingam*

As the name suggests, the objective of this phase is to creatively awaken the lingam. For many men the techniques used here can be so pleasurable as to bring them close to ejaculation. It is important to delay ejaculation here, however, in order to experience the full breadth of the lingam massage and its potential for truly deep sexual fulfillment. If you are close to ejaculation, give your partner a clear sign so that he or she can slow down or stop the stimulation, and instead distribute your energy throughout your entire body.

The giving partner can also press the *jen mo* point and vibrate the perineum with a fist. Apply pressure during your partner's inhalation, and remind him to relax during exhalation. He should continue to breathe deeply into his pelvis, with breaths that may become gradually more intense.

1. **Around the clock:** The lingam is resting on the belly and pointing toward the belly button; this is the 12 o'clock position. Use

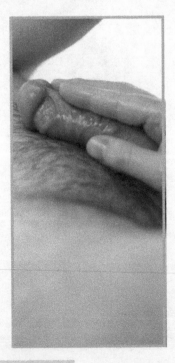

Phase 5: Awakening the Lingam

your right hand to gently stroke the lingam from base to tip, with your left hand gently pulling back the foreskin if your partner is not circumcised. Then move on by one hour, with the lingam now pointing at 1 o'clock. Again stroke the lingam from the base to the tip. Continue until the lingam has returned to the 12 o'clock position. In the 5, 6, and 7 o'clock positions, your hand will envelop the lingam entirely. Remain for a moment in the 6 o'clock position— this feels especially good when the lingam is soft or semi-erect.

2. **Gate of consciousness:** Gently pull down the foreskin and touch the area under the glans, the "gate of consciousness." This spot corresponds to our third eye, which is the origin of our visions. The nerve endings here are extremely sensitive. Gently massage this area in circular movements using your thumb and plenty of lubricant. While doing this, use your other hand to play with your partner's nipples or stroke his body.

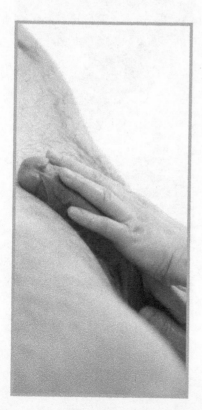
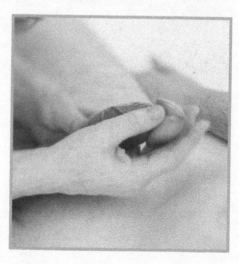

3. **The small delight:** Use both thumbs to massage to the left and right of the frenulum (the small band that holds the foreskin in place), in opposite directions, moving up and down on the lingam. This very sensitive spot corresponds to the heart chakra and the female clitoris. A nice variation: rub the skin of the frenulum between your thumb and index finger.

4. **Rainbow journey:** Place your hand over the glans like a hat and massage the lingam in the hollow space of your palm by moving it forward and back. In this way, the ball of your hand massages the gate of consciousness. For many men this is an entirely new feeling of fantastic pleasure, and some will see (rainbow) colors while you do this.

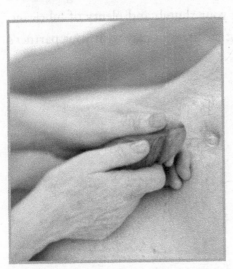
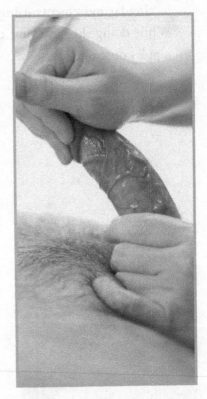

▲ *Phase 6: Riding the Wave*

In the sixth phase, which I call "riding the wave," the recipient learns to ride his own pleasure like a surfer rides the waves of the ocean. The massage giver maintains the role of attentive partner, ensuring that the recipient's pleasure builds, but is diffused just before ejaculation by the techniques described above. It is very important for the recipient not to be stressed or tense in this phase. If an ejaculation is inevitable, then enjoy it fully. Perhaps you will be able to delay ejaculation in the next lingam massage. If your arousal does not climb toward climax right away, then ride a smaller and gentler wave. The important thing is to fully enjoy your body and your sensations, accepting what is. If you remain conscious of this, then you will find over time a rhythm that matches your sexuality. Your breath can become quicker and deeper during this phase, and you can use your powers of imagination to circulate it through the Microcosmic Orbit.

1. **Merry-go-round:** Envelop the lingam with both hands and circle them in opposite directions. Move your upper body forward and back in sync with the movement of your hands, so that your whole body is involved in giving this massage. This can also include

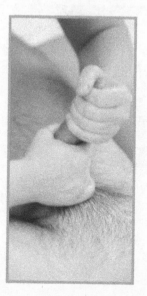 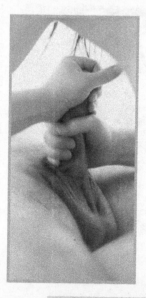

Phase 6: Riding the Wave

moving your pelvis forward and back. This rocking motion helps to guide your hands up and down on the lingam. When done well, this stroke can feel to the recipient like riding a merry-go-round.

2. **Healing stroke:** With the lingam resting on the stomach and your fingertips pointing toward your partner's feet, use the ball of either hand to glide down along the underside of the lingam (the side facing up when the lingam rests on the stomach), guided by the "gate of consciousness" (see page 143). In lingam reflexology this area corresponds to the spine. This stroke can be repeated several times—it feels pleasant and does not cause excessive stimulation.

3. **The big U:** While one hand continues the healing stroke, the other hand makes a movement like an upside-down large U from the knee across the perineum, up toward the stomach and the heart, then down to the other knee. This stroke distributes sensual-erotic energy in the body and connects the sexual center with the heart. As the recipient, let your sexual energy flow from your hips to every part of your being.

4. **Rocking the lingam:** With your partner's lingam resting on his belly, take the lingam between your two flattened palm—as though you were making a sandwich. The balls of your hands rest on the

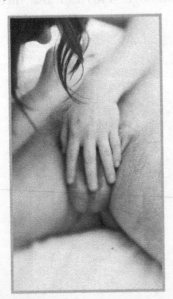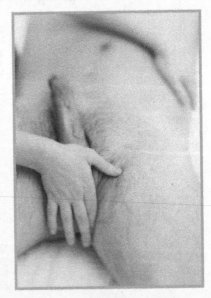

glans, and your fingers point toward your partner's feet. Moving your hands in alternate directions, slide up and down the lingam, varying your strength and speed. Use the back of your lower hand to also massage the lower abdomen. This is a favorite exercise for many men. Use plenty of oil or lubricant!

5. **Belly circles:** While doing a healing stroke with one hand, use the other to awaken the lower abdomen. To do this, massage your partner's belly in circular movements—first clockwise, then counterclockwise. Let your hands find a rhythm together.

6. **Generating fire:** Once the lingam stands upright, you can rub it between your hands the way you would rub a stick to make fire. Massage the lingam down to the base and then back up all the way to the tip. This stroke creates strong friction, which is why it is important to use plenty of oil. The friction creates a warming fire of empathy and vitality in the magical wand. You can alternate this stroke with the "rocking the lingam" stroke above.

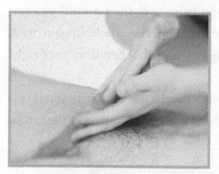
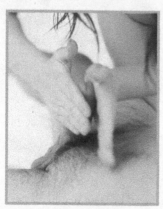
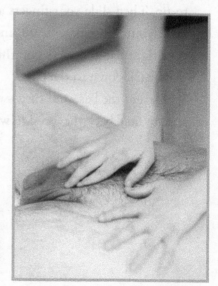

Phase 6

7. **Heart-genital bridge:** Use the lower part of your left arm to stroke from the pubic bone to the chest and back down to the pubic bone again, making sure to keep your wrist loose. This creates a connection between the heart and genitals. Use the other hand to perform the healing stroke or a more intense massage of the lingam, depending on whether you wish to build up or maintain energy.

8. **Carpe diem:** As you stroke the lingam in the direction of the heart, carefully stroke the testicles in the direction of the feet. Remember that the testicles are very sensitive at this point: pay close attention to your partner's face to gauge when his pleasure begins to feel like discomfort.

9. **Lingam tango:*** Sitting between your partner's legs, make yourself as comfortable as possible. Apply sufficient oil, then use your left hand to gently pull back the foreskin and hold it at its base. Hold the lingam shaft between the index and middle fingers of your right hand. Run your fingers up along the sides of the shaft from base to tip. Then slide your fingers and palm over the tip until you can bend your wrist downward and embrace the whole lingam with your right hand, fingers pointing downward. Then slide your right hand back down to the base.

   Rest at the base and then switch hands: use your right hand this time to hold back the foreskin while your left hand dances the tango.

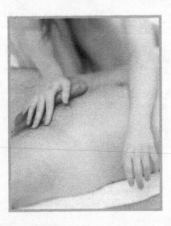 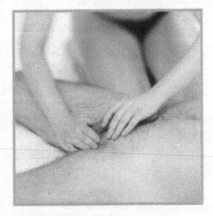

---

*This wonderful stroke was taught to me [Michaela] by Deva Bhusha.

The index and middle fingers of your left hand run up along the sides of the lingam shaft until you reach the tip, then slide your palm over, turn your wrist downward, and envelop the whole lingam as you slide down to the base. Rest there and then repeat the tango with the right hand. This stroke requires a little practice to learn; for that reason, you may want to practice it first on a dildo or a banana. But the practice is worth it for the pleasure that this stroke brings.

10. **The twist:** Pull back the foreskin with one hand and hold the lingam at its base with the other hand. Use this hand to massage the lingam in twisting motions up and down. Use plenty of oil and cover as much of the lingam as possible with the massaging hand. Breathe in rhythm with your partner. If you are receiving this massage, collect your energy as you inhale and relax as you exhale.

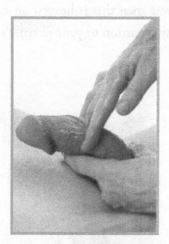
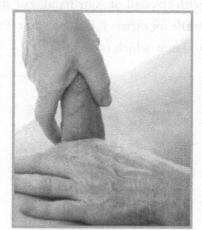
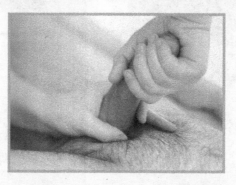

11. **Vibrating the root:** Vibrate the perineum as described in phase 4: Make a fist and press your knuckles gently but steadily against the perineum. With your other hand gently pull the scrotum upward, so that you can place your fist directly underneath it. Begin vibrating your fist. You can do this quite strongly and for a long time. If you are using your right hand to vibrate and massage the perineum, you can use your left hand to strongly massage the inside of the right thigh to the perineum. Then change hands—have your left fist massage the perineum, while your right hand massages the inside of the left thigh.

12. **Ringing bells:** Make a ring with your thumb and index finger and grasp the scrotum where it connects to your partner's body (ring grip). Use your other hand to make circling movements on the scrotum, scratch it lightly, touch it with your fingertips, and massage it with the ball of your hand. For some men this is heaven on earth, while for others it is unpleasant. Pay attention to your partner's face to know which is the case.

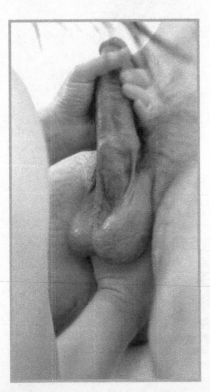
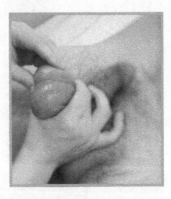
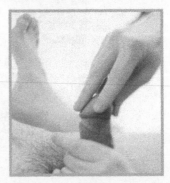

13. **The lemon:** Use one hand to pull back the foreskin. Use the other hand to massage the glans as if you were squeezing a lemon, using your fingertips to twist from top to bottom. This grip is done mainly with the fingers. Make sure not to exert too much pressure, as this can quickly become uncomfortable. As an alternative you can glide your fingers back and forth along the back edge of the glans.

14. **Spider legs:** Use one hand to pull back the foreskin and hold it at its base. Bring the five fingertips of your other hand together and very gently touch them to the glans. Slide your fingers lightly from the glans toward the base, until the your palm is resting on the glans. These movements should feel as gentle as spider legs.

15. **Twist and shout:** Combine the "twist" described in step 10 on page 149 with the "lemon."

16. **Lake of peace:** Use your left hand to massage the "lake of peace" between the nipples, while stimulating or holding the lingam with your right hand. This creates a connection between the lingam and the heart.

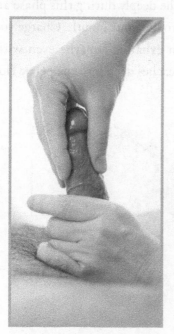
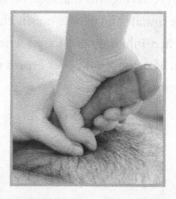
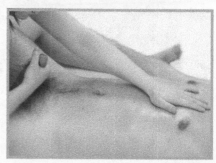

▲ Phase 7: The Finale

The seventh phase, the finale, is about steering the "wave" your partner is riding toward a climax. This is done by slowly building it up and consciously guiding your partner's energy from the root of his third eye to the gate of consciousness using the "Amsterdam" stroke. This sexual energy is then connected to his heart, before it is finally released in a climax of his choosing.

Every lingam massage should always be completely open to the experience of orgasm, with or without ejaculation. After thirty-two minutes or more of genital stimulation and "riding the waves," men reach a different state of mind. At this point, a full-body orgasm is possible, with or without ejaculation. The decision whether to ejaculate at this point or to use the Big Draw or "implode" by contracting the PC muscle is fully up to the recipient and should not be judged by his partner. All alternatives are welcome. It is, of course, interesting to try what one knows the least, which is usually an orgasm without ejaculation.

When receiving this massage, breathe deeply during this phase and, if you like, inhale and exhale noisily through your mouth. Charge yourself up when inhaling and let go when exhaling—maybe even with a deep sigh. Make sure that your breath reaches deep into the pelvic floor, to your root.

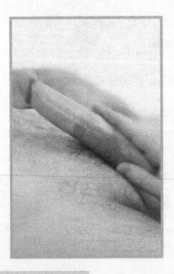 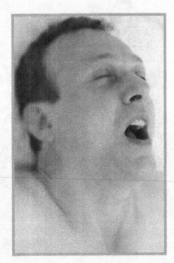

Phase 7: The Finale

1. **Generating fire:** When the lingam stands upright, rub it between your hands as if you were rubbing a stick to make fire. Massage the lingam down to the base and then back up all the way to the tip. Use plenty of oil, as this stroke generates strong friction.

2. **Heaven phallus:** One hand envelops the lingam and glides upward along it from the base. The other hand follows. In this way, the hands encourage phallic energy to rise up to the heavens. This is one of the few strokes where the foreskin is pushed over the glans. As always, speed and pressure can vary. Use plenty of oil, and be particularly careful not to trap and pull any hairs.

3. **Root phallus:** Both hands alternate in gliding down the lingam from top to bottom, returning the phallic energy to the root. Note that this is only pleasant with a full erection!

4. **Dance of the hands:** Cross your hands as if in prayer around the lingam and let them dance. Glide up and down while using your thumbs to simultaneously massage the "gate of consciousness" of the lingam—the area on the underside next to the frenulum. This is very arousing and the secret climax of the massage.

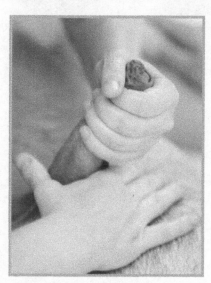
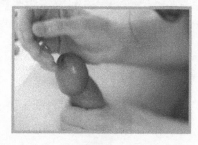
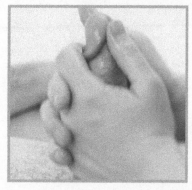

Phase 7

5. **Amsterdam:** If you are sitting beside your partner at this point, use one hand to vibrate the perineum and place the fingers of your other hand on your partner's third eye, forming a bridge between sexuality and spirituality. Conduct energy through your hands. If you are sitting in front of your partner, you probably won't be able to reach the third eye on his forehead. In that case, simply point toward it and remember that energy will follow your attention.

6. **Lake of peace:** Use your left hand to massage the lake of peace between the nipples while using your right hand to stimulate or hold the lingam. This stroke supports the sex-heart connection.

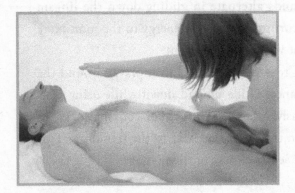

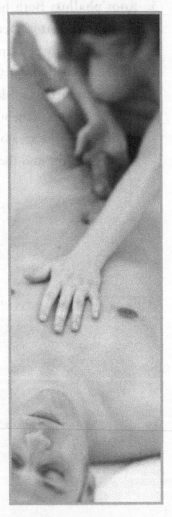

Phase 7

7. **As he likes it:** Massage the lingam the way your partner likes it. Ask him. With this last arousing stroke you invite your partner to a climax—with or without ejaculation—or to a gentle closing.

8. **The Big Draw:** If you are receiving a lingam massage and would like to end with the Big Draw, give your partner a signal so that he or she ends the massage before you ejaculate. Take a few quick and deep breaths, followed by three slow and deep ones. This will make your Big Draw stronger. Inhale deeply and tense your entire body: fists, feet, legs, arms, stomach, shoulders, face. Maintain this tension with your breath held for as long as possible, then let go completely and relax.

   If you have been giving a massage to a partner who signals that he would like to practice the Big Draw, you should now stop touching him. Cover him with a cloth or towel and sit quietly beside him. In this way he can concentrate fully on himself and the energy in his body. During and after the Big Draw it is important that the man be alone for awhile. Don't jump up immediately and walk away, however, or you'll miss the most important part of the feeling. Instead, remain present to witness your partner's completion without interfering in his physical and energetic system.

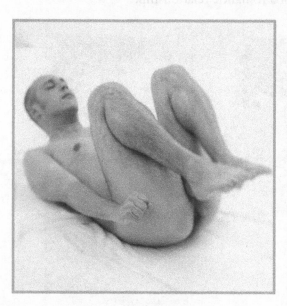
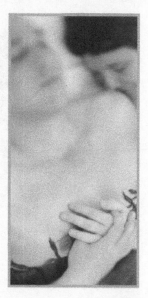

Phase 7

▲ Phases 8 and 9: Feeling and Farewell

The eighth phase is the phase of feeling, in which emotions that were released during the lingam massage can unfold. During this time, body and psyche process the information that was released and transform it into consciousness. Many men report trance-like states, intense emotions, prickling sensations, and the perception of colors or smells. After this, the massage giver can end the massage with a gentle hug or a brief touch to the heart or head.

The ninth and last phase is what I call "farewell." This phase rounds out the joint experience of the massage giver and the receiving partner. Here both partners can talk about any issues that come to mind, and ask questions of one another about the massage. Perhaps the receiving partner wants to briefly relate some of his experiences, or the giving partner wants to ask how a particular stroke was received. After this, the lingam massage session is over. Both partners can leave the room grounded and with clarity.

In our AnandaWave practice, each interaction is clearly defined and has a definite end. This is of course not the case if the lingam massage is given in the context of a romantic relationship.

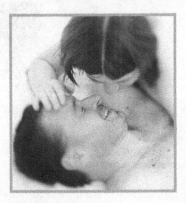
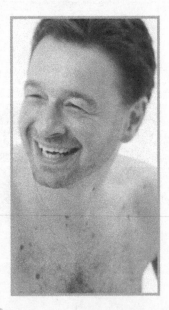

Phases 8 and 9: Feeling and Farewell

CONCLUDING THOUGHTS ON LINGAM MASSAGE

By Michaela

The compilation of strokes that make up the lingam massage was created by me and my partner at AnandaWave, Gitta Arntzen. We developed it based on our experiences in massage practice and in teaching our seminars. The individual strokes come primarily from the previously mentioned sexologist Dr. Joseph Kramer, from Andro Andreas Rothe, the head of the first German tantra institute (Berlin's Diamond Lotus Lounge, founded in 1977), from Margo Anand, founder of the Sky Dancing Institute in California and Europe, and from Deva Bhusha, a tantra masseuse at Sinnes-Art in Dresden, Germany.

Even though the sequence presented here makes sense as a whole and was developed after careful reflection by Gitta Arntzen and myself, it is important to note that the lingam massage should under no circumstances be a set program. It is much better to follow the phases of the massage and pay close attention to what the recipient needs at any specific moment. The massage presented here offers a broad range of different lingam massage techniques that can be mixed and matched in a creative and playful manner.

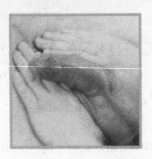

4
The Blessings
of
Anal and
Prostate Massage

Up to now we have focused mainly on the visible and known parts of male sexuality and in doing so have gone step by step into greater depth. Looking now at anal and prostate massages, we will enter an area that is new territory for most people. As we saw above, it is possible to massage the prostate via the perineum. However, a more direct approach, which has a more lasting effect, is to massage the prostate via the anus. An anal massage opens two pleasurable areas for men, each of which is worthy on its own of being discovered and included in our sexual experience.

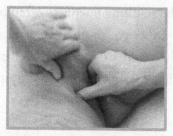

ANAL MASSAGE: SOURCE OF AROUSAL AND LETTING GO

Our entire pelvic floor is a source of deep arousal and sexual sensations. This is why it makes sense to include the anus as a normal sexual zone in both male and female sexuality in spite of the many taboos. If we really want to know ourselves in all our sensuality and sexual strength, we need an open anus, not a constricted one, and a strong, flexible pelvic floor. If we enjoy arousal in the "front," but block it in the "back," we will have an incomplete experience of arousal and of our sexuality. For this reason, a relaxed anus during a full erection is very important for male sexuality.

Just like any other muscle, the anus can be sensitive and allow sensual feelings to permeate, or it can close itself off and block them. If the anus is tense, sexual energy is not able to flow sufficiently throughout the body. Instead, it remains blocked and limits our sensitivity and receptiveness.

In our practice we notice that many men have a closed, hard anus and are too fixated on their erections. They lack the ability to let go, to enjoy themselves, and to be receptive. In these men, the penis does its part, but we feel that the soul of the man is not responsive, not present. Unable to fully perceive themselves or their partners during sex, such men often complain of sexual problems like premature ejaculation, difficulties achieving or maintaining erections, or a lack of sensitivity to stimulation. Digestive problems, hemorrhoids, and even impotence are often the result of tensions of the pelvic floor area, especially in the anus.

If the anus has an opportunity to relax through an extensive and loving anal massage, the resulting openness often brings men into contact with their ability to let go, to open their hearts, and to connect with themselves and the world around them. With a relaxed anus, men are more able to experience deeply human and deeply sexual feelings.

The Anal Problem

Developmental psychology suggests that children begin to discover their anal sphincters at age one-and-a-half or two. This is an important moment in the life of a child, when for the first time it understands: "I can let something go, but I can also control it and keep it in." On another level this means: "I can say 'yes' or 'no.'" Often, however, this important discovery is destroyed by overly strict hygiene training. The child is supposed to learn as quickly as possible to master the sphincter and become potty trained. However, each time the potty is not nearby and a child feels the need to defecate, he or she begins—completely against the natural impulse of simply letting go—to control the sphincter with full effort. But since the nerves necessary for this are not yet fully formed, the child's body becomes tense all over: in the buttocks, the back, the belly, and the jaw. It is even reflected in the breath. In this way the first blockages develop.

This "anal tension" can develop into two different character traits: a child who learns to control the sphincter with all its might becomes "anal retentive"—overly precise, perfectionist, and pedantic. A child who simply gives up in resignation becomes unable to hold things together later in life, becomes chaotic, disorganized, with a lack of concentration—a person without drive.

In both cases people are holding back one part of their arousal experiences, freezing it to "survive." Since in the first phase of childhood the libido is very much anchored in the anal region, everything that influences the child from the outside becomes associated with it—be it limits, power, excessive fear, or excessive care.

This experience and our internal attitudes toward it often manifest over the course of years in an unconscious ongoing tension of the pelvic floor. That is why it is important for both our general well-being and our sexual health to be able to consciously feel and relax the pelvic floor, including the lingam and yoni as well as the anus.

However, no other part of our bodies is linked to as many prejudices as the anus. In our day-to-day life we tend to perceive it as a necessary body opening and an embarrassing and dirty area. Many people have never reached inside their own anuses, since this area almost as a matter of course causes feelings such as disgust or shame. Anal intercourse thus remains one of the last taboos in many people's sexual lives, and anal dreams are often kept from the partner. Men who would like to be stimulated anally fear being seen as gay or "female." Our society's moral stance leads many of us to close our anus until it hardens and keeps our sexual energies from flowing freely.

For this reason we often begin our seminars with questions that are deliberately provocative.

- ▲ Is it really necessary to include the anal area? Isn't that dirty, gross, perverse, abnormal, and sexually obsessed?
- ▲ Are we allowed to feel arousal and pleasure in every part of our bodies, or only in some?
- ▲ Is it not enough to get to know our lingam and yoni and play with them? Does it have to be anal?

Following these questions we then consciously begin to transform these negative images, and learn to live in the body with all its openings, celebrating the godly in our anus. In this way we quickly see that there are no areas that are dirty or gross, and that we can use the anal region especially to allow more consciousness, arousal, and pleasure into our lives. With this new experience and knowledge, our relation to the anal area changes enormously. When we then ask our participants what they feel in the anus, they often answer: relaxation, pleasure, width, peace, deep connectedness, softness, letting go. This gives us the answer to our first question: "Yes, that's exactly why we do it."

Honoring the Anus

Tantric philosophy teaches us that all our body's openings are holy and that god can be found even in our excretions, since god is everything and encompasses both our light and our dark aspects. It is very important for our humanity that we do not exclude the dark side of the godly. In the West we are very fixated on the positive and the light and usually want to have little to do with the dark sides of our beings. We want to love only the "beautiful" parts of people and either want to change the "negative" parts or exclude them. But if you fixate only on the light parts of life without embracing and accepting the dark, you cannot let go, and will remain "anal retentive" your whole life.

A clear need to control one's surroundings can suppress spontaneous feelings and block emotional expression, as well as one's strength in life. Unexpressed emotions like aggression and anger then get stored in the body, and can later give rise to illnesses and difficulties with orgasm.

Once we learn to have a loving and respectful relationship with the anus, it changes our entire being, and makes us more loving and gentle, both toward ourselves and toward others. In this way we integrate, honor, and release the "asshole" within us and thus—as if in a fairy tale—turn a frog into a prince.

Acceptance and Desire

Once we learn to accept all aspects of our sexuality, sensuality, and arousal, we can approach the anus with respect and acceptance. In that case, even a single anal massage can suffice to resolve deep-seated feelings of disgust. Disgust is always linked to a moral judgment. If I take a finger and enter someone's anus while keeping this judgment in my head, I will likely only increase the feeling of disgust. But without a moral judgment, an anal massage will bring me into contact with the deepest parts of another person—with his limits, extremes, joy, pleasure, and pain. It creates a communication on a very deep level, confined within a very beautiful, respectful frame that creates an aesthetic and comfortable atmosphere. In this way the anal massage becomes normal, is integrated into our understanding, and causes the moral judgment to lose its power. Something that I understand with acceptance loses its disgustingness.

I can well recall my own first anal massage. I did not have an easy time since in my anus there were literally gorges and cliffs that had to do with abuse of power, impotence, helplessness, shame, and incredible anger. This initially led me to not want to burden anyone with my anus. But once I overcame these initial hurdles of letting go, energy began to flow; my heart and the deep experience of spirituality became tangible, and I experienced for the first time an absolving feeling: my anus was part of me! It was my garden of paradise.

It is thus very much worthwhile to bring the anal area out of its dark shadow of repression into the light of acceptance.

THE PROSTATE AND THE G-SPOT

In men, the special nature of anal massage is increased by a further aspect of deep arousal and enjoyment: the massage and stimulation of the prostate, the place of physical strength and connectedness. Aside from the benefits to health and potency that this massage brings, the prostate massage opens an entirely new way of experiencing sexual arousal, completely different from the arousal we experience through the lingam.

Just as most women report a deeper, fuller, and more lasting orgasm when stimulation of the clitoris is complemented by a massage of the G-spot, an extensive prostate massage in men also leads to a deep and lasting orgasm. The healing opening that is possible on all levels during prostate massage allows sexual energy to spread throughout a man's body and being.

Men say the following about the prostate massage:

▲ "The arousal increases greatly. Every touch is much deeper."
▲ "Openness, softness, being taken."

▲ "The whole pelvic floor and anal area feel warm and pulsate—somehow charged with energy."

▲ "My orgasm with a prostate massage is not quite as intense, but much wider and more all-encompassing."

Many men report that a prostate massage helped them experience a deeper feeling of sexuality and build better contact with their own anus and pelvic floor. Feelings like joy, arousal, softness, pain, horniness, and sadness surface. Others report feeling "female" or "exposed."

An anal and prostate massage connects men deeply with the receptive, "female" side of their sexuality, which many are not used to. They experience for the first time what it is like to spread their legs and allow something to enter them; they learn what it is to be penetrated, to be "taken." With this experience, men are able to combine two aspects of their sexuality that appear to be at odds with each other.

▲ A full erection, if accepted, honored, and respected brings men in touch with their powerful strength. Combined with the qualities of power, courage, potency, strength, stamina, and readiness for action, the phallic strength is a source of life and a symbol of masculinity.

▲ As men learn how to connect these qualities with their "female" attributes of openness, devotion, fullness, and tenderness, they can use their phallic strength as an expression of love and for the benefit of all life. They connect their sword—the warrior within—with their internal woman, a being of love and devotion. Sword and rose become one.

The Yin and Yang of Our Sexuality

Clitoral orgasms are often described by women as sharp, short, and strong—like an explosion. These descriptions are very similar to what men say about orgasms that occur exclusively via the lingam—that they're strong, short, explosive, usually limited to the genital area. This type of orgasm allows us to experience the yang, more "male" sensations of our sexuality.

On the other hand, women variously describe their G-spot orgasms as "wide," "connected," "deep," "enduring," and "very connected to the heart." This is similar to a male orgasm that has been primarily triggered by the prostate: "enduring," "touching," "deep," and "carried." This type of orgasm allows us to experience the yin, the more "female" sensations of our sexuality.

Stimulating both the clitoris and G-spot in women, and the lingam and prostate in men, helps men and women to feel more whole in their sexuality. Women connect with their "male" aspects and men with their "female" ones. This melding of yin and yang allows us to become whole and healthy.

THE SPIRITUALITY
OF THE PELVIC FLOOR

The pelvic floor, anal region, and the prostate are governed in our body's consciousness by the first chakra, also called the root chakra. The central themes of the first chakra are life and survival, birth, material security, fundamental needs, original energy, grounding, and stability. From this perspective, the first chakra can be seen as the basis on which all the higher refined potentials rest.

The physical processes of taking in food, digesting, and excreting, which are part of the first chakra, in many ways correspond with our emotional perception processes. In eating, digesting, and excreting, we take things from the outside into our bodies, process them, and then return them to the world in the shape of expressions, acts, or creations.

The massage of the pelvic floor and the buttocks create a relaxed depth. This brings us into contact with our connection with the earth, and brings stability into our lives. If the first chakra is brought into harmony, for example through an anal or prostate massage, men can lead their lives in harmony with the laws of nature and rooted in deep feeling. Professionally and financially they will live in security, enjoy their material well-being, and be generous in giving and taking.

Yogis and tantric practitioners describe a latent energy potential that rests within us at the lower end of our spines; it is a kind of original energy. This so-called kundalini is represented by a snake. You can use your PC pump (see page 36), to encourage this energy to rise upward along the spine through each of the chakras. This changes your state of consciousness.

ANAL AND PROSTATE MASSAGE AND THE ABILITY TO TOUCH

An anal and prostate massage touches the being of a man in a very immediate way. On a physical level we cannot go any deeper, cannot penetrate any further. For this reason, it is important to see an anal massage as opening and entering the most holy temple of a man. This helps us to be respectful and loving in the massage. Opening the anal canal can initiate healing processes on the physical and spiritual level, independent of awakening the kundalini energy.

If the anal area is very tense and the touch is new, an anal massage can initially be unpleasant, or even painful, for the recipient. The tissue in this area is often hardened, but can be loosened through a slow and conscious touch. A healing relaxation during the anal massage can also cause hot spots in the anal area. Finally, many people have stored sexuality, aggression, and life strength in this area, which from here can be brought back and released into conscious experience.

The opening of the anal canal should thus be a slow and respectful process. This requires a clear, attentive and protected space within which men feel accepted and supported. Honoring all parts of a man and unconditional respect are essential in this regard.

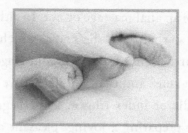

ANAL AND PROSTATE MASSAGE
STEP BY STEP

As in lingam massage, here too it is important to carefully prepare for the massage because a clear and respectful atmosphere is often decisive for the success of an anal and prostate massage.

As the recipient, mentally prepare for the massage by celebrating a sensual cleansing ritual. This can be a lot of fun. I usually use a scented shower gel and a little Vaseline and take a shower.

After you have thoroughly cleansed your whole body, take the shower head and crouch down. Then take a finger with a little Vaseline and apply it to your anus, gently opening your anus until your finger is inserted. Open your anal canal in the same way. Then pull the anus opening a little to the side and hold the showerhead with the water stream against the anus opening. Let the water flow into your anus. Keep the water in your canal for a little while and use your pelvic and stomach muscles to move it back and forth a little. Then press the water, with all its "contents" out again. If needed, repeat this two to three times.

It is also recommended that you avoid foods that cause flatulence—like beans or cabbage—for one or two days before the anal massage. This often makes access to your inner temple much easier.

If you suffer from hemorrhoids, it is better to be treated by a doctor first, since these can be painful. Nonetheless, I have in the past received an anal massage while suffering from minor hemorrhoids; it was possible because my partner avoided stimulating the injured spot. Decide for yourself how strong your hemorrhoids are and whether you would like to receive an anal massage or not. In either case talk to your partner beforehand so that he or she knows which areas to avoid.

As the giving partner, make sure that your fingernails are cut short before exploring the anus, and that you don't have any rough or sharp spots on your middle or index fingers. Now begin, just as with the lingam massage, by preparing a loving, pleasant and warm room (at least 80 degrees Farenheit) with nice fabrics, fresh flowers, candles, and sensual background music. Prepare a massage area in the center of the room (or the part that you consider the center) with all the tools that you will need for this massage (for example feather, fans, cloths, furs, massage oil, lubricant, a bowl with hot water, washcloths, a small hot-plate, Vaseline, and perhaps latex gloves).

Prepare each other just as I described the preparation for the lingam massage on page 119.

Wear a nice kimono, a sarong, or a bathrobe. As the giving partner, take the lead and sit down with your partner in the massage area so that the two of you are facing each other.

Notes for the Person Giving the Anal and Prostate Massage

Be fully aware that you will be touching the innermost parts of your partner in this massage. Open yourself to this deep encounter with all your heart. Remain in your center and accompany this ritual with love and your full presence of mind. There is nothing to achieve or to force. Be aware that often the smallest touch in the anus can cause a volcano of feelings in your partner.

If you encounter blockages or areas of hardened tissue, these spots can become physically warm. Remain on them as long as it doesn't cause your partner pain to do so, and simply wait to see whether the temperature lowers and the spot returns to feeling normal. If so, old memories, experiences, or physical blockages have been resolved. This can cause strong feelings in your partner, including grief, pain, anger, happiness, or laughter. Accompany your partner in this too. Remember: there is nothing to do other than to simply and lovingly be present. Continue to enter into communication and ask your partner whether the pressure, speed, and movements are pleasant and whether you should change anything.

During an anal and prostate massage, your partner will frequently lose his erection. Instead, he may be experiencing an entirely new dimension of his sexuality, which he will learn to bring into harmony with his phallic strength. Even men without erections are deeply satisfied and feel sensually touched in a prostate massage. Acknowledge this and don't try to change anything.

After the massage, allow yourselves enough time to talk about the experience. Look after yourself and your own needs after an anal and prostate massage.

Notes for the Person Receiving the Anal and Prostate Massage

A new and exciting journey is about to begin, and it is completely normal that this unusual expedition into the innermost part of your temple may initially cause some discomfort, shame, or fear within you. Take note of this lovingly and make the conscious decision to dare this new healing step.

Open yourself to this new experience and remain fully present in the here and now. Continue breathing into your pelvis and register what is happening. Be like a father watching his child at play: without judgment, without forcing, without expectation—simply feel, observe, and breathe, and let yourself be taken care of.

During anal and prostate massage it is very important that you communicate with your partner and tell him or her whenever you need a break from the intensity of the last touch. Tell him or her when it is good to continue, to change the speed, to massage more in the back or the front, or simply to end the massage. It can also be very helpful to communicate feelings that may arise within you. This can be very liberating. Try it!

After the massage, allow yourselves enough time to talk about the experience.

There are several ways of carrying out an anal and prostate massage, which I want to describe in detail at this point. In this context, it is important to know that arousal spreads from the front to the back, which means that before a prostate massage (not anal massage) the lingam should be stimulated to a pleasant degree of arousal. Before all massages is always the honoring of the Shiva as described on page 120. Then there are the following options:

▲ Anal and Prostate Massage—Option I

Begin with honoring the Shiva and the preparatory full-body massage, with your partner lying on his stomach. Make sure to finish by extensively massaging the buttocks and entire pelvic area. Then ask your partner to get on his hands and knees and crouch behind him.

1. **Full moon** (*for the recipient*): Make yourself as comfortable as possible in this position. Let your head hang down, bend your back with pleasure and present your buttocks by pushing them in the air and consciously relaxing your pelvis. A poet once said, "When a man is on all fours, the butt shows its full beauty, it rises like the moon." In this position your anus relaxes and your pelvis opens. It also makes it very easy for the massaging partner, sitting or crouching right behind you, to reach everywhere—an important precondition for a good anal massage.

2. **Body massage:** Make sure that you can reach everywhere, and massage your partner's entire body from this position: his back to the neck, the buttocks, the legs. Then put on your gloves. This sequence is always described with gloves, since being able to massage with gloves is an art in itself. If you know each other well, the massage can also be done without gloves.

3. **Around the rosette:** Take enough Vaseline or balm and lovingly apply it to his rosette. Get a sense for what it feels like and then use your fingers to circle along the rosette and the outer sphincter.

4. **Opening:** Keep pulling the rosette very gently from all sides. Then

gently increase the pressure on the sphincter by continuing to press your finger gently a little bit into the opening. Now you can get a very good feel for whether the anus is wide, relaxed, and open or hard, tense, and closed. Take your time.

For the recipient: Feel this touch and be present and awake. If you feel resistance, take deep breaths. Contract your sphincter and then consciously let go. Ask your partner to continue massaging the outer sphincter a little while longer.

5. **Entering the anal temple:** When you feel that the anus is ready, soft, and open, use your middle finger to enter the anus gently but steadily, with your palm facing up. Make sure that the entry is conscious and gentle, but not too slow. The sphincter is programmed to press everything out of the anus. It will begin to contract as your finger enters, which can be unpleasant and a little painful. As soon as your finger has gone past the sphincter, these contractions will reduce.

6. **Rest in the center:** When your finger is all the way in the anus, remain there without moving and give your partner a little time to get accustomed to the feeling.

7. **Anus clock, first half:** Now begin massaging the entire anus extensively from the inside, using circling, clockwise movements. Picture the rosette as a clock and begin using the left middle finger to massage gently from the back to the front at 12 o'clock. Then move on to 1 o'clock and continue on until you have reached 6 o'clock. If the sphincter begins to contract, you will be able to feel the strength of this muscle. If this happens, rest where you are and wait until the contractions stop again. Remain in contact with your partner and ask him whether your touch is pleasant or whether he'd prefer you to change anything.

8. **Changing fingers:** At 6 o'clock, gently and slowly pull out your left finger and insert your right finger, well lubricated with Vaseline. While doing this you can use the thumb of your right hand to take off the left glove, leaving your left hand free again to massage the

entire body. You can also use it to now massage the lingam, the perineum, and the testicles, again using plenty of lubricant.

9. **With both hands from behind:** At 6 o'clock, use the middle finger of your right hand to gently press down relatively far back; you will be able to feel the prostate. It will feel like a round, hard rubber ball. If you want to massage it more intensively from this position, you should first use the left hand to lovingly massage and stimulate the lingam, including also the perineum and testicles in your touch. Once you note a light arousal, begin with a gentle prostate massage while continuing to gently stimulate the lingam.

10. **Awakening the prostate:** You can massage the prostate with small circling movements or with in-and-out movements. Perhaps you will be able to insert a second finger into the anus. Ask your partner and let him give you feedback. Can you feel the prostate growing slightly and becoming more noticeable to the touch?

    For the recipient: Can you feel your prostate? How does it feel? You may want to share your feelings with your partner.

11. **Anus clock, second half:** Use the middle finger of your right hand to thoroughly massage your partner's anus clockwise from 6 to 12 o'clock with small circling movements. When you return to 12 o'clock, very slowly pull out your right finger. Let it rest on the outside of the rosette for a little while, then ask your partner to lie down on his stomach again. Cover him and give him a few minutes to feel the effects of the experience.

    For the recipient: Be entirely present and feel the effects of this intense journey by listening inside your body and observing what is happening there.

12. **Frontal full-body massage:** Ask your partner to turn around and continue the full-body massage on the front of the body, as described on page 131.

13. **Lingam massage:** Begin with an extensive lingam massage, using the strokes described on pages 142, until your partner is nicely aroused.

14. **Return to the prostate:** Pull a glove over your right hand, apply Vaseline to your middle finger, and enter gently but steadily into the anus. Massage the prostate, which you can now feel at the top, slightly to the left of you.

15. **Both hands from the front:** Now combine the lingam and prostate massage. Continue switching between the two and closely observe your partner and get feedback from him.

16. **Finale:** Choose the finale that is best for your partner. Ask him! Then cover him with a cloth and conclude the massage as described on page 152.

   For the recipient: Feel within yourself to decide which finale would be best for you at this point.

   ▲ Perhaps you want a conclusion with or without ejaculation through a combination of lingam and prostate massage.

   ▲ Perhaps you want your partner to conclude the prostate massage and to reach your desired conclusion with a lingam massage.

   ▲ Perhaps you want your lingam to simply be held while the finger in the anus continues to gently massage the prostate or simply rests there. Communicate your desires.

▲ Anal and Prostate Massage—Option 2

After honoring the Shiva, begin with a full-body massage of the front and back of the body as described beginning on page 127.

1. Continue with an extensive lingam massage (referring to the section on lingam massage) until your partner is nicely aroused.

2. Begin an extensive anal massage as described above with your partner lying on his back. It is not as easy from this position, but will be easier for both of you if you slide a thick cushion under your partner's buttocks.

3. Conclude by combining the lingam and prostate massage, again as described above; then find a good conclusion.

▲ Anal and Prostate Massage—Option 3

After honoring the Shiva, begin with a full-body massage of the front and back of the body as described in the section on lingam massage.

1. Continue with an extensive lingam massage (using parts of the lingam massage described earlier) until your partner is nicely aroused.
2. Ask your partner to turn around and to get on all fours as described above.
3. Begin an extensive anal massage as described above.
4. Then ask your partner to turn around once more. See whether it is possible for you to keep your finger in his anus as he turns around.
5. Then combine lingam and prostate massage, again as described above. Together find an appropriate conclusion.

It makes sense to try all three options. In this way, the receiving partner can find out which option works best for him.

NAMASTE

Experience Reports

~~~

The following experience reports of men were recorded immediately after I [Michaela] had administered a lingam massage to them. The reports are mostly recorded word for word, although I at times omitted passages of less interest to the reader, and at others paraphrased some statements in the interest of readability and clarity.

LINGAM MASSAGE WITH MICHAEL

Michaela: How are you?

Michael: I'm well. Very well. Nicely relaxed. Full of energy.

Michaela: Perhaps you want to tell me about the full-body massage before we talk about the lingam massage. What were the moments in which you felt really able to let go?

Michael: Actually right from the beginning, from the welcoming ceremony. Yes, that was a nice introduction to relaxation.

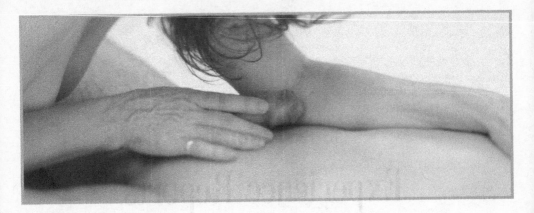

Michaela: What do you need to be able to relax?

Michael: No distractions. Very soft music.

Michaela: Do you prefer more slow movements?

Michael: It's all right for them to be quick and strong at times, but in general, yes, I prefer them slow.

Michaela: Does that make it more sensual?

Michael: In the case of strong strokes the intensity is very high, and you reduce some sensors to be able to deal with that, so it's less of a comprehensive experience in that way. But there, too, there were moments where the massage was strong and quick, but because they were preannounced and not sudden, I was able to anticipate them. That change was very pleasant, and it created a feeling of encompassing everything from toes to fingertips to my hair.

Michaela: What elements are very important to you? What would you really miss if it wasn't part of the massage?

Michael: Oh, I can't say. The massage was wonderful as it was.

Michaela: Okay, I'm happy to hear that. Then let's talk about the prostate massage. Can you tell me how the prostate massage felt for you and what you need during it? What happens to you during the prostate massage?

Michael: The prostate of course is a highly erogenous zone. The intensity that is created there is very different than in the lingam, something very deep. I couldn't orgasm through a prostate or anal massage. But it gives me a feeling of depth and additional arousal.

Michaela: A different kind of arousal?

Michael: Yes. If I compare it to music, it's something like the bass, which you normally hardly even notice, but which makes music that much fuller.

Michaela: Then we continued with the front and with the lingam massage. Did you experience different qualities in the strokes I used?

Michael: Yes. What I noticed especially is how the lingam was at first included playfully in the massage of the front of the body. I had the feeling that the lingam massage was really a part of the massage. And yes, I liked that very much.

Michaela: So you were already a little warmed up for the lingam massage?

Michael: Yes, it aroused me.

Michaela: And that arousal lasted for the duration of the massage?

Michael: Yes, it did.

Michaela: Oh, that's nice. How did this arousal feel?

Michael: A light arousal, like an appetite.

Michaela: Then I began with the lingam massage by pressing into the lingam (lingam shiatsu). How did that feel? I was pressing quite hard.

Michael: Yes, but I like that every time. Sometimes I like strong pressure, at other times I prefer a lighter touch, I don't know why that is.

Michaela: Afterward I stroked the lingam into the four directions of the sky, forward and backward.

Michael: Yes, that had a relaxing effect.

Michaela: Is it important to you that the lingam massage is prepared carefully, or could you imagine taking your lingam without applying oil first and just getting started?

Michael: No, that wouldn't be as nice—it has to build up gradually. It's not about having an orgasm in five minutes, but rather about enjoying the massage. And that's why for me it is really important to have it be a gradual process.

Michaela: So you are able to fully enjoy the slow progression?

Michael: It prickles sometimes, and I think to myself: "wow, now I could go up a level," but looking back I think I would regret it if everything had come to an end too quickly.

Michaela: So you enjoy holding the tension that is built up?

Michael: On the one hand there is the desire to give in to the arousal quickly, on the other the wish to enjoy everything very slowly and to prolong the experience. That is part of what creates the tension. Most men like both, I think. But both doesn't work—one has to choose.

Michaela: By now you have had quite a bit of experience with lingam massage. Is it based on that that you say: "It's much better for me if I can prolong the experience?"

Michael: I'm here to enjoy myself. If I want to have it quickly, I can do it myself at home, as they say—on the toilet or in the shower.

Michaela: What is the qualitative difference in the experience for you?

Michael: It is deeper, much more intense, with effects that last longer. It's also a different way to approach my sexuality. Otherwise it is all about stronger, faster, quicker. In the movies you see athletic fuck-machines that build up great speed and you start to think that that's what it's about. But at some point you realize, no, that's not what it's about. You learn to value a different perspective. And that includes things like this massage, just to experience what it's like when you take it very slowly and spend a lot of time. It is wonderful, even if it's hard at first. After some time you can completely let go and accept it as it is.

Michaela: What helped you in being able to withstand this tension?

Michael: Hmm, somehow you learn it. It's like having a partner who gets you to enjoy the slowness, the pleasure. And then you notice that this is good for you and you start doing it yourself. It's not about just a quick act, but about enjoying it slowly and for a long time.

Michaela: So you're saying you're able to celebrate this for yourself as well?

Michael: Yes, you can do wonderful things by yourself too, if you take your time and enjoy yourself. But if you are able to focus only on receiving, it adds another quality.

Michaela: Because the stimulation comes from outside?

Michael: Because you don't have to be active yourself, but can concentrate fully on the feelings.

Michaela: We started riding the waves in the lingam massage. There were moments when you said: "Oh, please stop, don't continue, or else . . ." I sometimes got the feeling that the waves were really going far up. How are you able to feel yourself enough to be able to ride these waves? How do you make sure not to ejaculate too early?

Michael: I'm sorry, I just feel that, I can't explain it.

Michaela: I don't think that everybody could do that.

Michael: I think most people are able to feel where they are on this path, whether they are far up or not yet.

Michaela: So if ejaculation happens at 100 percent, you would be able to tell when you're at 50 percent?

Michael: Yes, I can judge at any time where I'm at. And you just have to make sure to break before passing the point of no return.

Michaela: How?

Michael: By giving a sign, saying "Stop. No more, or at least not like this!" And then you can begin to approach that point again.

Michaela: How do you delay ejaculation when you have sex with your partner? Is it intuitive?

Michael: Very slow, gentle movements.

Michaela: Do you have the feeling that it has something to do with consciousness? How much you enter the moment and how much you feel what's happening?

Michael: It does have to do with consciousness and the interaction with my partner. I feel where she is at, and I know that she doesn't like this in and out, but prefers the slowness, and that's what I do. Most men can do slow for a long time.

Michaela: Sometimes I meet men that have many images in their head. Do you have such images that you know, if these come now, it'll get difficult?

Michael: No, I don't have fantasies to reach orgasm. With my partner I don't always orgasm. There are days when I'm not in top form. But I don't worry about it. It doesn't happen often, but from time to time. On the other hand: if I accidentally get close to 100 percent too quickly, I think briefly about my taxes to engineer a break.

Michaela: Were you comfortable with simply lying there during lingam massage and receiving? That's different from being with your partner, where you are an active participant.

Michael: I really enjoy being able to do nothing at all and simply receive. Yes, it's a real pleasure.

Michaela: Is it not really difficult just to lie there?

Michael: It's not so much the touch of the lingam, but the more accidental touch in between. That can be quite a lot, I don't need fantasies or images, I don't have to do anything, it's on the whole and by itself very stimulating.

Michaela: It's nice to hear you talk like this. It sounds very fulfilling.

Michael: Yes, and I'm really full now.

Michaela: Your energy was relatively high, and then we included the prostate. How was that?

Michael: On the one hand, it added to my arousal, but on the other hand, I noticed that my erection decreased a little, and it took a little while until it was back as before. But in general it was a more intense, encompassing feeling of arousal.

Michaela: They say that it helps men get in touch with their receptive, female side. Did you feel that way?

Michael: A little. It had to do with opening. I had the feeling of being completely exposed. I don't know what that would be like with someone I didn't like.

Michaela: Does it feel different when you have an orgasm and the prostate is included in it?

Michael: Today I had the feeling that it was more intense. But from my experience I know that that isn't always the case.

Michaela: You didn't practice the Big Draw, but I know that you have done it before. How is it for you when you practice the Big Draw instead of ejaculating?

Michael: I usually don't get this intense feeling after the Big Draw. I haven't really warmed up to it.

Michaela: So it's more that you contract your body during the Big Draw, then let go, without anything really happening after that?

Michael: That's right.

Michaela: Men can experience orgasm and ejaculation separately . Have you experienced that?

Michael: I think it is true, but I couldn't describe an exercise that would be able to accomplish that. I felt that in part a few times, the feeling that my body was tense and energy-rich as in an orgasm, but without the Big Draw.

Michaela: You can always do the Big Draw, including during inter-course. Simply contracting the muscles and then letting go again—so it doesn't always have to be that "big." But you have experienced at least in parts the feeling of orgasm without ejaculation?

Michael: A little. I have an idea of what it's about.

Michaela: I have often seen men that can ejaculate without having an orgasm, and then on the other hand there are orgasms that last a long time. What does that depend on?

Michael: I think it depends on the time that one had before. If you have a very fast quickie, you might have a great ejaculation, but that's about it. After two minutes the whole feeling is over. And if you take a lot of time and gradually increase and get into your arousal, if you take a lot of time and don't give in to the impulse to have an orgasm as quickly as possible, then it's like an explosion that affects you for a long time. That's a difference.

Michaela: What are the most important elements of a lingam massage for you?

Michael: First, the normal massage. I call it the normal massage because it doesn't include the genital area, or includes it only in passing. I need that to relax fully. And then I like it that there are such different elements that are part of the massage later. If you masturbate, you know what you like, which leads to less experimenting. But when you receive the massage it includes strokes that one wouldn't have thought of. There are variations that cause certain sensations. Some things you may like less, others really get under your skin in a good way. It's like a colorful salad in which there are all these very delicious things. It's the mix of it all. That's why I can't say that I would like to have this or the other element.

Michaela: Thank you. What would you say to someone who would really like to experience a lingam massage?

Michael: It is a chance to learn something about yourself. Because you can focus entirely on discovering your own sexuality. If you are with a partner, it is an interaction—which also has a special quality—but you are always half with yourself and half with your partner. In a lingam massage, I am entirely with myself, I don't have to look after somebody else, how they are feeling, whether I am going too fast or too slow. I can concentrate fully on myself, and in that process, discover and learn more about myself. And that has positive effects on sex with a partner, too.

Michaela: What positive effects?

Michael: There is a better quality. I learned not to give in to the impulse to ejaculate quickly. Once you have experienced how nice it is to delay it, then you internalize that. You don't have to think about it, it's clear. Slow, steady, that's not even a question. Conscious sex.

Michaela: Conscious sex. Very nice. That is a good last word. Thank you very much for this interview.

LINGAM MASSAGE WITH
BERND

Michaela: How do you feel after the massage, Bernd?

Bernd: Very good. I am really energized, my whole abdomen feels warm and charged. It is still vibrating. Vibrating and pulsating. And the Big Draw at the end really distributed the energy throughout my body. The feeling during the prostate massage was completely different than during the lingam massage. Especially on the hands and knees. At first the prostate hurt a little, and I noticed that I wasn't used to this.

Michaela: Yes, when I was there with one finger, I first massaged the right side very extensively and then the prostate.

Bernd: That's right. Exactly. Were you there with two fingers or with just one?

Michaela: With just one.

Bernd: Really? When you left I had the feeling that there was a certain back and forth. It tickled a little too.

Michaela: Yes, I once discreetly changed fingers. I have to massage the left side with the right finger, otherwise I get a knot in my arm.

Bernd: The moment of leaving and reentry was very pleasant for me, an entirely new experience. I've never had it like that, the focus, time, and preparation. I really enjoyed having the rosette lotioned and massaged with so much love. I really enjoyed that and was able to relax deeply and coordinate my breathing.

Michaela: Yes, I had the feeling that that was working well. When you were exhaling your anus opened wide, and I was able to slide inside it without any problems.

Bernd: One has to let go in a very conscious way for that.

Michaela: Yes, that's right—that really is the moment where one decides to let go, and that's not entirely easy . . .

Bernd: At the very beginning I noticed that I briefly contracted the muscle. It was a kind of reflex.

Michaela: The anus has a reflex that wants to press everything out that is or wants to be inside. That's why the slow penetration of the anus isn't that good, and can in fact be very painful because the reflex is working against it. That's why I asked you to inhale and then slid in pretty quickly when you exhaled.

Bernd: Then the reflex only came once more. Instead, I felt the impulse to let go.

Michaela: Do you want to tell me about the massage as a whole? What you liked, and what you didn't?

Bernd: The way you held me at the beginning gave me a feeling of comfort and safety, which I also found very erotic. I had an erection right away. And the way you opened my kimono and slowly reached past my chest, I really liked that. When I closed my eyes briefly and you invited me to breathe, that immediately brought me into myself.

Michaela: I felt that. You went with me very nicely.

Bernd: I was able to really let go when we were breathing together. I also liked how you played with my hair and how you used both of your hands to stroke my bottom from bottom to top. That was very nice, especially on the front of my body. And also on the stomach, and down the legs across the tops of my feet. That really took the pressure off my legs.

Michaela: What do you need to be able to let go, to feel safe, and to feel sensually touched?

Bernd: The feeling of being carried, of being held. These small gestures, the way you held my hand or pulled me toward you. And the feeling that I am welcome, the safety of having the other person be 100 percent there. I had that feeling the whole time with you. Yes, that also makes it erotic. It's special and beautiful to be able to enjoy, and not have to do anything. And of course the sensuality. It's also nice to feel your body, your legs, a little of your breast on my body and to feel that it's not only hands, but every once in a while also other elements that are very erotic and sensual. I lie there and think: is it the leg? Or the butt? That stimulates my mind.

I also liked the change between strong and gentle, playful passages. One moment it's a deep massage, then a very erotic one, and then the gentle strokes. Every once in a while strong, having your thumb go into something hard and tense, that feels liberating.

Michaela: How is it for you to remain passive during a sensual massage? To really do nothing at all, which is less common for men?

Bernd: When I first started receiving lingam massages, it was a bit unusual, and I remember asking myself: "I can just accept this without doing anything?" But when you really allow this to happen, it's a very beautiful thing. And it's all the better the more one is able not to have thoughts like "I should have an erection now," or "I should ejaculate now." This massage invites one to recognize that it is about touch and feeling. I am allowed simply to take, to allow myself to be presented with gifts.

Michaela: Then there is the other topic for men in the massage, which is to close the eyes. I personally think it's okay for men to open their eyes every once in a while and have a look, since this is important for men and makes some things easier. I think men are much more visual than women. How did you find this?

Bernd: I had my eyes closed during the massage, right from the beginning, since I noticed that watching is distracting for me. It's definitely erotic to look every once in a while, but it immediately brings you into your head. When you have your eyes open, it's harder to go inside yourself. That's why I think it's better to, for example, feel a leg and wonder: "Was it the butt?" I find that much more erotic than to look and see what's really happening.

Michaela: And about the individual steps of the lingam massage. At the beginning I massaged a lot along the perineum. How was that for you?

Bernd: Very good. You can do that for a long time if you want. And in general that's an area where you can also massage strongly.

Michaela: Don't you think it scares men when the focus at first isn't on the lingam, but on the perineum?

Bernd: Well, you began with the lingam shiatsu and that was a great preparation. But a personal thing: when you were gently shaking the lingam back and forth, before it was erect, the head was rubbing against the hairs, because I am circumcised. That was not so stimulating, but that's of course a matter of personal preference. But that was really an exception.

Michaela: Yes, I think the head is a very special subject. What do you need so that one can touch your head in a good way at some point?

Bernd: I really liked the lingam shiatsu, also the clockwise stroking (healing stroke). That's a good preparation. Mainly not to go for it right away—really the steps as you did them. Sometimes I also think it depends on the day, like the clitoris—sometimes the head is not so sensitive, but sometimes a direct touch is too strong. Especially the juicer (the lemon) was not so pleasant for me in past massages, because it was too strong, too much stimulation. But today I really enjoyed it.

Michaela: And then, after the root, I did the clockwise stroking, and you liked that. Then I included the whole body in the massage with the "big U" and had the feeling that you also enjoyed that, especially when I include the perineum and really go into it.

Bernd: Yes, with the strokes. And the gentle strokes in general. The circling on the stomach with the arm up and down (heart-genital bridge)—I really liked that, because it had something opening, freeing, and resolving.

Michaela: Did you get the feeling that with the strokes up and down the energy was getting distributed throughout your body?

Bernd: I can't say that I felt energy traveling up and down my body, but it was like a deep breath, like an "aaahh." It brought an opening, a widening of the chest.

Michaela: And then I gently rocked the lingam, and then came the "fire."

Bernd: I really enjoyed that. It could even have been stronger.

Michaela: That's true, but honestly, I didn't really dare go any stronger, because that's often the point at which men ejaculate.

Bernd: I'm relatively good at giving a sign early enough, so it's not like "oops, here I come." But I didn't say anything, also because I didn't know what else was to come. Then, during the second prostate massage while I was lying on my back, it was very intense, and afterward everything felt very broad and wide within myself. And it was nice to have the lingam touched during that massage.

Michaela: Well, I had a really beautiful feeling, that's why I continued for such a long time without feeling funny or thinking "oh no, it's getting boring, I should stop." It was very meditative and beautiful; there was a lot of energy. The lingam too had a lot of energy, even though the erection had gone. It was nice to massage like that; I really enjoyed it.

Bernd: And it could have been even longer. It wasn't like, "All right, I'm not getting an erection, better to stop now." No, it was actually very nice to continue feeling your touch. And when you asked, "So, do you want to keep going?" for a moment I asked myself: "Okay, can you get an erection again?" I put myself under some pressure and then thought, "No it's not going to happen anymore." Also, I had to pee and then I can't get one up anyway, that's how it is for me. And it wasn't necessary anymore, feeling-wise. I feel very energized now.

Michaela: I know that from yoni massage too. When I receive an anal massage and at the same time there is one finger on the G-spot and one in the anal area, and both are stimulated at the same time, I feel a very strong arousal that has nothing at all to do with a normal orgasm. Where the orgasm feeling disappears completely, but a different arousal surfaces that has a completely different quality that nourishes and fills me.

Bernd: Exactly. That's how it felt for me the second time. During the first prostate massage I was very aroused, and really enjoyed having you stimulate my lingam a little in between. That was really great and I was very aroused.

Michaela: Can you describe that in more detail?

Bernd: It was really great, really great. Also the feeling of being "fucked" as a man, to be penetrated. Also from the fantasy, the feeling. Yes, I found it very erotic to open myself like that.

Michaela: Did you feel a little exposed, especially on your hands and knees?

Bernd: Yes, a little. But that's not negative at all—it was something erotic. I don't have a problem with that, but I could see how it would be difficult for some men to present themselves in that position.

Michaela: At first it's new and feels a little foreign, to get on your hands and knees. In those cases I will take note of that and make sure to provide a clear framework and clear directions: "Okay, now get on your hands and knees and make yourself comfortable." There are those who say: "No, I don't want to." But that's more rare.

Bernd: Yes, it's important that you are sensitive to this and very clear about it.

Michaela: Is there anything else you want to tell me?

Bernd: In general I think it's really important to have plenty of time. That makes it easier to let go and to enjoy oneself. Two-hour massages are best. Also to try the prostate massage. It's good to experience that once; it is something very special.

Michaela: Well, that's a good conclusion. Thank you for this extensive interview.

Bernd: My pleasure.

LINGAM MASSAGE WITH WOLFGANG

Michaela: What motivated you to come to AnandaWave for a lingam massage, and how do you feel now?

Wolfgang: I came because of a very strong sexual insecurity. At the end of the massage I felt that I was back in touch with my sexual strength and security, even if not 100 percent. I was very touched when I felt that my strength, confidence, and consciousness came back, which I used to take for granted.

Michaela: Can you tell me how you reached that point?

Wolfgang: Being understood as a man by the woman who was massaging me. That she understood what was going on inside me. Before this strength came, there was a moment when my body let itself go. At first I was rather stiff and tense, and there was little I could do about it.

Michaela: At the beginning of the lingam massage?

Wolfgang: Yes. And then I could feel my body letting go as it developed trust that it would not be mistreated. Mistreated in quotation marks.

Like a car engine. If you change the spark plugs, the engine won't run right anymore. And during the exercises before the massage, I could feel my body growing more confident: "This woman won't do anything that will irritate me, but will treat me with care and love." The body grew to trust the hands that were touching it. I consciously tried not to force anything, not to focus on getting an erection or becoming aroused, but simply to give in to what I felt and what developed in the massage. And that created a deep touch, and when the kundalini rose up, certain elements of my normal sexuality suddenly came back. For example, that my kundalini came back, that it flashed up, and so on.

Michaela: Can you explain what it's like for you when the kundalini "flashes up" as you describe it? What exactly happens inside you then?

Wolfgang: I just call it kundalini. I don't know whether that matches what the Indian yogis are referring to. I experience it as a blockage in my pelvis loosening and then energy rising up through my spine and shaking my whole body. Not a shaking that I cause, but a shaking that happens within me. And if I allow that to happen, I experience a kind of connection with a flooding of light, with a gaining of strength. There's a different type of presence that permeates me. A strong presence. I call it "Shiva appearing in me." This "appearance of Shiva" is what connects me to my masculinity; it is there and wants to show itself through me. I find that an incredibly beautiful experience.

Michaela: Yes, that sounds very beautiful. When you knew that you would receive a lingam massage, did you have certain thoughts, expectations, or images?

Wolfgang: Well, at the beginning I felt pretty unsure, to be honest. Also, because it was the first time in my life that I was receiving a lingam massage from someone other than my partner.

Michaela: And how did you deal with that feeling of insecurity?

Wolfgang: At first I was tense and felt cold. And when I am tense and cold, then it's often a sign that there's something that I don't want to feel. Subconsciously I had the wish to be very relaxed and happy during the lingam massage. Then I asked myself: "If I felt something, what would it be?" And then I felt a sexual frustration from my past. I decided to tell you how I felt at the moment, and I also had the courage to say that I was feeling sexual inadequacies and was stuck in a midlife crisis. I didn't expect a solution at that moment, but to be able to describe how I felt without having it be judged was necessary for me to open myself to the lingam massage. And when you said that it didn't matter whether I had an erection or ejaculation or not, it created for me an open space in which anything and everything could happen. And the first thing that I learned in the massage was trust. To trust your hands and my body, and to basically bathe my body in this trust, that it would get what was good for it.

Before the massage I was aware that I had grown used to a certain finickiness. When my girlfriend touched me, almost any touch felt unpleasant, because I was afraid of being touched in the wrong way. At first, I also felt this discomfort during the massage, but then I told myself: "It's alright, Michaela knows what she's doing, just relax." When you spread my thighs and moved something, I could feel my pelvis opening and feel energy flowing inside it. That was the point at which I felt sexual energy again.

Michaela: I often take up what is present there, what is being offered by the body and the person himself. And I got the very strong feeling that it was more important to be gentle, to hold and accept, and that sexual energy was less important.

Wolfgang: Yes, for me that was exactly the right starting point. I allowed myself my sexual insecurities and they were caught, and that was very important for me as a man. And then the soft way of experiencing sexuality. It was important to begin with releasing lots of tensions. I felt like dough that was being kneaded.

Michaela: Many people want to skip this step, but the body first has to feel full and safe. Then we can live both sides, the soft and safe, and the sexual and phallic.

Wolfgang: I now think that the sexual problems I have with my girl-friend are partly because of me. Before I saw the causes as lying only with her.

Michaela: You didn't have an erection during the lingam massage, and it's not necessary, since it's possible to enjoy the massage to a very high degree even without one. But I could think that it would make a dif-ference.

Wolfgang: I would say that it's more sexual when I have an erection, more horny. But the feelings still went very, very deep, even without an erection. I had deep emotional experiences that often switched between tears and laughter.

Michaela: I felt that a very gentle approach would be best, not necessar-ily the fiery part that is sometimes present in a lingam massage.

Wolfgang: Yes, that's true. When the lingam is not erect, it's better to have a gentle touch. I think that the lingam has a lot to do with reflex-ology zones, because a lot of images came up during the course of the massage. There were also very strong spiritual moments, where I some-times cried and sometimes laughed. So the erection wasn't necessary to have those experiences. When the lingam is full and erect, it goes more toward the outside, when it is not erect, more toward the inside, the depth. You could compare the full lingam to the sunny and the other with the moon side. They are simply different aspects.

Michaela: That is a very nice statement. When we as women are con-fronted with a lingam that is not erect, it causes a lot of insecurities. I know that from my own experience. It's really nice if women can better understand what is happening in a man. That it can go into depth, and that a nonerect lingam prefers a gentle touch. Thank you for this.

Wolfgang: The lingam is really a teacher, for both men and women. And we should leave it to the lingam whether it wants to be erect or not. But we men have learned that it should function. I prefer not to function but to be human, authentic, honest, and tangible, rather than trying desperately to build up an erection. That's just stress, and in the end it prevents me from being truly intimate with a woman.

Michaela: Was there something during the lingam massage that was unpleasant, or something that you would have wanted?

Wolfgang: There were two things that were not entirely perfect for me. One was that the underside of the testicles are very sensitive, especially where the epididymides are. I don't want to be touched there. Making a ring around the testicles from the top is wonderful. But touching, especially the right testicle and epididymis—that I don't like. The second was during the "small delight"—I found that a little too strong. But I told you that and you adjusted your grip.

There were a couple of things that were really great. One was spreading the thighs and the vibrating of the perineum—even though it wasn't phallic it felt really good. I also liked that very normal movement that I know as a man when the foreskin is slid across the glans. I find that very arousing. And it was important to me that you continued to stroke and distribute the energy throughout my body.

Michaela: How would you like your testicles to be touched? Can you tell me something about that?

Wolfgang: I enjoyed it when you pulled down my testicles with your grip; that was great. When the testicles are pulled down, they normally want to move up again and somehow that feels really great. The other thing I like is when they are scratched and prickled, I find that stimulating. In general, I find that touching the testicles is more erotic when I am already aroused, when I am more sexual. And it's a real turn-on to have the lingam and testicles be stimulated at the same time. Touching the testicles then is nice, stimulating.

Michaela: How was it for you when the lingam massage was over and you were feeling inside yourself?

Wolfgang: My whole body was vibrating, I know and love that feeling. And I finally felt energy in my body again. The massage also made me more aware again of what I need. In day-to-day life, I sometimes have a tendency to put my own needs last, or not to feel them so strongly. What was important afterward was being held, that you didn't leave abruptly and leave me alone. I had the need to be held, to be close to someone. And then I noted, yes, now I can gradually let go, but I needed my own time so that it didn't happen too abruptly.

Michaela: Thank you very much for this talk.

Afterword

~~~

By Joseph Kramer

I read the first pages of the book *Lingam Massage* by Michaela Riedl and Jürgen Becker and am thrilled. At this point I would like to recount how I myself arrived at lingam massage.

In 1979 I was training to be a massage therapist, with the desire to offer men and women new ways to experience their bodies. While other masseurs were focusing on treating back pain or chronic tensions, I wanted to awaken the body's tissues with my hands and to bring each client as deeply as possible into a state of physical pleasure.

One day after I had finished a very good massage the man on the table asked me: "Didn't you forget an important part of my body?" I was astonished and irritated, since to me, my calling to awaken bodies didn't seem to have anything to do with touching the penis. As the man was leaving my studio, he said, "I feel hurt by your massage." I was speechless. Was it possible that I had hurt the man by not touching his penis?

Over the course of the next weeks I asked myself whether I myself had been sexually hurt during my massage sessions. I came to realize that I was carrying trauma in my genitals. And it was possible that I was transmitting my own injuries during each massage session.

If I wanted to include the penis massage in my sessions, I would have to know more about it. Unfortunately I did not have access to teachers of erotic massage, so I began my research on my own body. I experimented with different types of touch, sometimes strong, sometimes gentle, slow or quick, in rhythm with my body or my breathing. By leaving behind my usual erotic paths, my entire life became less defined by routine. I felt a new freedom and began to use what I had learned on my own body in my massage sessions with other men. In the last twenty-five years I have taught lingam massage to more than fifteen hundred men and women around the world.

In 1991, on a trip through Europe, I visited the massage therapist Isa Magdalena in Amsterdam. For two hours I was lost in the best body massage that I had had in years. Then she surprised me with the question: "Would you like me to include your penis in the massage?" I nodded. Her penis touch was good, almost too good. She touched my penis in exactly the way that I do it. When she had used a series of massage techniques on the most sensitive part of my penis, which I call the "gates of consciousness," I asked her where she had learned to touch a penis like that. She said: "A friend of mine learned this last year from an American." I waited until the end of the session to tell her that I was this American.

The lingam massage contributed to the creation of a new profession in California, sexological bodywork, which has been officially recognized since 2003, and which plays a central role in genital massage. Today there are sexological bodyworkers around the world.

Joseph Kramer, Ph.D., is Professor of Somatic Sexology at the Institute for Advanced Study of Human Sexuality and is the founder of The New School of Erotic Touch. He can be contacted at www.eroticmassage.com or www.sexologicalbodywork.com.

Notes

<hr style="width:20%">

CHAPTER 1

1. See Michaela Riedl, *Yoni Massage: Awakening Female Sexual Energy* (Rochester, Vt.: Destiny Books, 2006), 37, figures 1.17 and 1.18.
2. Ian Kerner, *Mehr Luft für ihn: Was Männer beim Sex verrückt macht* [More Air for Him: What Drives Men Crazy During Sex] (Munich: Goldmann Publishers, 2007), 41.
3. Robin Baker, *Sperm Wars: Infidelity, Sexual Conflict, and Other Bedroom Battles* (New York: Basic Books, 2006).
4. Webpage of Todd Shackelford and Aaron Goetz: www.toddshackelford.com
5. Dr. Wolfgang Beier, *Potenzprobleme erfolgreich überwinden* [Successfully Overcoming Potency Problems], Audio CD (Regensdorf, Germany: Verlag für Positive Lebensgestaltung, 1998).
6. Frank Sommer, *VigorRobic: Increased Potency through Specific Fitness Training* (Düsseldorf: Meyer & Meyer, 2007), 30 [in English].
7. Ute Michaelis, *Beckenbodentraining für Männer. Harninkontinenz und Erektionsstörungen mindern und überwinden* [Pelvic Floor Training for Men: Alleviating and Overcoming Urinary Incontinence and Erection Dysfunction] (Munich: Urban and Fischer Verlag, 2006), and Benita Cantieni, *Tiger Feeling: Das sinnliche Beckenboden-Training für sie und ihn* [Sensual Pelvic Floor Training for Her and for Him] (Munich: Südwest Verlag, 2003).
8. William Alexander and Culley Carson, *Erectile Dysfunction* (London: Mosby, 2003).

9. Michael Pfreunder, *Schon wieder zu früh . . . ?* [Come Too Soon Again . . . ?] (Stuttgart: Verlag Integrative Weiterbildung, 2005).

10. S. Ebrahim et al. "Sexual intercourse and risk of ischaemic stroke and coronary heart disease: the Caerphilly study," *Journal of Epidemiology and Community Health* 56 (2002): 99–102.

CHAPTER 2

1. Osho (Bhagwan Shree Rajneesh). *Das Orakel der Meditation* [The Oracle of Meditation], Sutra 48 (Cologne: Innenwelt Verlag, 2001), 106.

2. See Mantak Chia, *Tao Yoga der inneren Alchemie: Das Geheimnis der Unsterblichen* [Tao Yoga of Inner Alchemy: The Secret of Everlasting Life] and *Fusion der fünf Elemente* [Fusion of the Five Elements] (Munich: Heyne Verlag, 2006). Originally published in English as *The Taoist Soul Body: Harnessing the Power of Kan and Li* and *Fusion of the Five Elements*.

3. Julie Henderson, *Das Buch vom Summen* [The Book of Humming] (Bielefeld, Germany: AJZ Druck und Verlag, 2007). Originally published in English as *The Hum Book*.

4. Mihaly Csikszentmihalyi, *Flow: Das Geheimnis des Glücks* [Flow: The Secret to Happiness] (Stuttgart: Klett-Cotta, 2007). Originally published in English as *Flow: The Psychology of Optimal Experience*.

5. Jörg Stolley-Mohr, *Der Body-Flow—Kontakt zum intuitive Körperbewusstsein* [Body Flow: Contact the Intuitive Body Awareness] (Mullheim, Germany: Auditorium Netzwerk) [Auditorium Netzwerk is an online shop for CDs and DVDs].

6. Ulrich Clement, *Guter Sex trotz Liebe* [Good Sex despite Love] (Berlin: Ullstein, 2006).

7. Stephen Wolinsky, *Die dunkle Seite des inneren Kindes* [The Dark Side of the Inner Child] (Stuttgart: Lüchow, 2004). Originally published in English as *The Dark Side of the Inner Child: The Next Step*.

8. Douglas A. Bernstein and Thomas D. Borkovec, *Entspannungstraining: Handbuch der 'progressiven Muskelentspannung' nach Jacobson* [Relaxation Training: Guidebook on the "Progressive Muscle Relaxation" according to Jacobson] (Stuttgart: Klett-Cotta, 2007). Originally published in English as *New Directions in Progressive Relaxation Training: A Guidebook for Helping Professionals*.

About the Authors

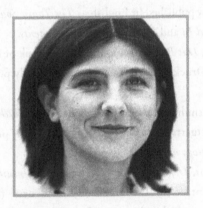

MICHAELA RIEDL

Born in 1968 in Straubing, Bavaria, Michaela Riedl began a tantric yoga course following a university degree in music. During the course of her yoga studies she learned about the yin-yang massage, erotic massage, tantric massage according to Andro (of the Diamond Lotus institute in Berlin, Germany), and the yoni and lingam massage according to Joseph Kramer and Annie Sprinkle.

Touched and inspired by the healing effects of tantric massage, she developed her own massage style over the course of her professional practice. In partnership with others she opened the first tantric massage practice in Cologne, Germany in October 1996 and was responsible for developing its contents. Drawing on regular courses and research on male and female sexuality, she developed today's AnandaWave massage—a further development of classic tantra massage.

AnandaWave massage activates and stimulates the entire body in a dynamic and loving way, awakens sexual energies, and distributes these throughout the body. Special massage offerings focus on different parts of personal healing.

In August 2005, Michaela Riedl and Gitta Arntzen opened the tantra massage practice AnandaWave with seminar offerings on "room for sensual experience." Here, people searching for personal expression in the areas of sensuality, sexuality, and spirituality are able to individualize their experiences. Offerings include various massages, different massage workshops for men, women, and couples, as well as instruction and certificate courses in tantric AnandaWave massage. These are complemented by seminars about bodywork, meditation, and personality development. Lectures about female and male sexuality as well as events demonstrating the AnandaWave massage round out this program.

A new massage and counseling about "ways out of irritation" is aimed at those looking for loving and sexually enriching relationships to themselves or their partners. Themes can include "getting to know one's own female sexuality," "orgasm problems," "erection difficulties," "premature ejaculation," and "speechless in bed."

Sexual and communication counseling for individuals and couples underline the holistic approach of AnandaWave. These are offered together with Constanze Rinck, who is a systemic family therapist and communication trainer.

Since 2007, AnandaWave has advocated for sensual experience in the German council of tantra massage, especially in the area of education.

▲▲▲

In *Lingam Massage*, Michaela Riedl presents information from her many years of massage and seminar work, which she continues to develop with Gitta Arntzen and the team at AnandaWave. For further information contact:

AnandaWave—Space for Sensual Experiences
Michaela Riedl and Gitta Arntzen
Riehler Str. 23
50668 Cologne
Germany

Massage offerings: +49-221-1793511
Seminars and organization: +49-221-4208028

E-mail: info@ananda-wave.de
Websites: www.ananda-wave.de or
www.tantramassagen.de

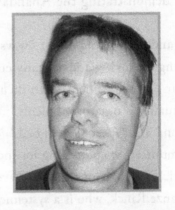

JÜRGEN BECKER

Jürgen Becker was a manager in a large company when a decisive experience markedly changed his relationship to sexuality and his own body: in 1989 he received a series of massages in postural integration (PI). The goal of PI is to free the body of frozen structures through deep touches and breathing and return it to its original vitality.

Even though the genitals are not touched during this bodywork, Jürgen Becker had a deep orgasmic experience during one of these sessions that greatly exceeded his "normally" experienced orgasms. In subsequent sessions these experiences were repeated. After this, he began to intensively research tantra, massage, and breathing techniques, trained as a life coach and counselor, and became a student of the spiritual master Osho.

Inspired by the book *Yoni Massage* by Michaela Riedl, he took courses in lingam and yoni massage in 2007 and 2008 with both AnandaWave in Cologne and with Pamela Behnke at Taste-of-Touch in Denklingen, Germany. The possibilities of lingam and yoni massage fascinated him, and he decided to write the present book *Lingam Massage* together with Michaela Riedl.

In the counseling practice that he operates with his partner near Munich, he accompanies individuals and couples through a dialogue therapy on their way to sexual consciousness and a fulfilling love life.

▲▲▲

For further information:
Klaus Jürgen Becker
Hauptstr. 28
82229 Seefeld
klausjuergenbecker@web.de

Index

Page numbers in *italics* refer to illustrations.

BOOKS OF RELATED INTEREST

Yoni Massage
Awakening Female Sexual Energy
by Michaela Riedl

Tantric Sex for Men
Making Love a Meditation
by Diana Richardson and Michael Richardson

Tantric Orgasm for Women
by Diana Richardson

Slow Sex
The Path to Fulfilling and Sustainable Sexuality
by Diana Richardson

Tantric Secrets for Men
What Every Woman Will Want Her
Man to Know about Enhancing Sexual Ecstasy
by Kerry Riley with Diane Riley

The Complete Illustrated Kama Sutra
Edited by Lance Dane

Healing Love through the Tao
Cultivating Female Sexual Energy
by Mantak Chia

Sexual Reflexology
Activating the Taoist Points of Love
by Mantak Chia and William U. Wei

Inner Traditions • Bear & Company
P.O. Box 388
Rochester, VT 05767
1-800-246-8648
www.InnerTraditions.com

Or contact your local bookseller